The Comprehensive Guide to Cancer Caregiving:

A Helping Hand for Patients, Caregivers, Family and Friends

C.L. UEBERROTH

For my Dad,
*Who faced cancer with the utmost strength and
faith,
Teaching me the lessons needed to survive grief.
You told me to remember you and think of you
from time to time, but I think of you everyday and I
wish I could have told you how life could never be
the same without you.
I miss you everyday and I love you.*

**For my family of caregivers, my mom and
sister,**
*Who pulled together in the battle of cancer that led
to this book's creation,
And who give me the strength to find my way into
each tomorrow.
I cherish you both and I love you both.*

For Dr. Hofstetter,
*Who gave us time & believed in my dad.
You are the best doctor I'll ever meet, who I have
undying gratitude for.
We were just one more patient's family you saw,
but to us, you are a hero.
Thank-you for your extraordinary care.*

CONTENTS

Introduction ~ Everyone Has A Story

Introduction ~ Everyone Has A Story

Everyone has a story to tell about the cancer diagnosis. It's never like the chicken pox or a sinus infection, where you see the doctor to diagnosis a problem you are already rather aware of. And often every person in a family has a different story to tell about the same diagnosis. My story of cancer starts with the mail. It blind sighted me on an idle Friday.

The mail arrived and life appeared fine. I was at my parents' house, a warm, rather ideal home in Orange County. The backyard still displayed the playhouse my dad built for Christmas some fifteen years ago, a beautiful barbeque with elaborate brick and tile work that he installed and a black bottom pool with a spa, slide and diving board surrounded by lush Hawaiian style landscaping. My Dad and I removed all the wallpaper in the home, sanded, textured and painted one summer while my mom and sister were at ballet camp. He laid the marble throughout the entryway, family room and kitchen and re-roofed the house. We teased and had competitive battles to determine whether he or my sister or I played his grand piano best. He loved his piano practically as much as his truck. His guitar was as dear as any of the tools that filled the garage where our "Tool Man" spent time building, creating and planning for the future. Our lives abounded with happy, laughter-filled dinners around the table my dad built, vacations throughout the country and teamwork. My parents placed my sister and me, our little family, above anything else and worked diligently to protect and nurture the family.

Until the mail arrived that Friday in October of 2003, the problems of my life consisted of tough mid-terms and traffic. The medical bills in my hand changed everything. I sliced open the envelope, curiously searching the insurance bill for a recent emergency room visit of my own. The bill caused my knees to buckle. Instead of my name next to the claim, my dad's name appeared column after column, next to one oncologist title after another. My eyes carefully studied: "Gastrointestinal Oncologist", "Radiation Oncologist", "Surgical Oncologist" and roughly the puzzle of the last month slipped into place.

Choking on a chip and an emergency room brought cancer into my life more realistically than the mail. My mom sent my dad to see the physician who treatment me in the emergency room. He needed a physical, she thought, and the doctor's business card read "Internist." She called one day and made an appointment with Dr. A., scheduling my dad for a physical. The receptionist gladly scheduled him for an appointment in a few weeks.

My dad arrived at the doctor alone for a routine physical.

"What's going on with you?" Dr. A asked.

"I'm here for a physical," my dad answered with a friendly smile.

"I don't do physicals, I'm a gastroenterologist," the doctor replied.

"I've got no complaints, I'm here because my wife scheduled me for a physical."

"Well, I'm not sure why they let her make an appointment for a physical, but since you're here and you have to pay for the visit, is there anything regarding gastroenterology I can address?"

My dad assured him there wasn't, but he pressed and questioned until finally Dad threw out, "I often get the hiccups when I start to eat."

By the end of the day he was scheduled for an esophagogastroduodenoscopy, more commonly known as an upper endospcopy, and we were cracking jokes at him, saying he was having surgery for the hiccups. As I held the insurance papers in my hand and cried, and my mind traveled back to the day after the procedure, things began to make more sense. Suddenly there were a thousand bottles on the sink consisting of vitamins, herbs and supplements, cabbage and other vegetables were being frantically juiced. And dad actually drank it! And I kept finding mom leaving uplifting notes for Dad. I asked a number of times, in a variety of forms, what was going on, but was convincingly and repeatedly told he had esophagitis and that was all. "Okay," I sarcastically quipped, "So you guys are expanding the business to include a health food store then?" My mom smiled nervously back.

One night haunts me. I walked into my dad's garage where he housed his office and found him playing the guitar. He usually played in the house. His eyes seemed glazed and emotion filled, but I was busy asking something. He said, before I turned to head back into the house, "I love you honey." My family openly showed love and affection, but this was out-of-the-blue.

I turned and replied, "Okay, enough of this, something is going on. What is happening? You and mom are acting so weird; tell me what is going on." He fought tears fiercely as he assured me nothing was going on.

"Why does the note on your desk say your mom's hero then?" I insisted.

He laughed to cover up the pain. "You know mom."

"Ya, I know mom, and that's just weird." But with one or another similar refutes, the conversation just ended. I guess they would tell us if it was serious, I assumed.

I stood alone in the kitchen that day, opening the mail. My Dad was out running his business and my mom sat watching my sister's tennis match. I erupted with emotion, growing completely hysterical. My dad arrived home and I hid in my room. It was too much to bear. As soon as my mom stepped through the door I cornered her and demanded, "What is wrong with Dad?"

"Why," she returned, looking panicked.

"Does Dad have cancer?" I sobbed.

"Hold on, let me go get him." He came in and the truth surfaced. That doctor investigating the hiccups found a tumor the size of an apple. All the new doctors called him "either the smartest man alive or money hungry," for investigating the hiccups. That day gastric adenocarcinoma bombarded our lives. Nobody would tell me the statistics, although they had to know I would head straight to the bio-medical library on Monday. They had the top surgical oncologist, medical oncologist and radiation oncologist and were playing the waiting game. They wanted to have all the information before horrifying my sister and me.

My dad said, "Why didn't you just come and talk to me when I got home."

"I didn't want it to be true," I shook with grief.

"It's going to be okay. We're going to take care of it. I've got a lot of living left to do. I'm going to be around for a long time. We have got great doctors, we're going to take care of this," he comforted me as I cried and cried in his strong arms.

Chemotherapy consisted of brutal inpatient twenty-four hours a day, seven days a week treatment. Radiation ran thirty days long, for two different courses of treatment. Surgery, one of the two most difficult surgeries performed in the nation, removed his entire esophagus, nearly half his stomach and the maximum number of lymph nodes. Surgery ran about twelve hours long and left him unable to consume water, food, or ANYTHING by mouth, for an entire month. Treatment came upon recurrence, entailing experimental runs on one drug after another, including two biological therapies. There were alternative treatments, conferences, enough cancer literature to stock a section at the library, multiple cancer hospitals, feeding tubes, pain medications, pain management, palliative care and hospice. Upon diagnosis of recurrence, we all stopped our outside lives, pulled together, traveled together, lived together, celebrated together and grieved together.

Everyday felt like a learning experience. Cancer has this learning curve about it that is difficult to keep up with: where mistakes can mean the difference between sickness and health, and life or death. I would sit in the medical center talking to people just diagnosed and feel sorry for all the learning ahead. It's like walking into a black hole: uncharted, unknown, unfamiliar, and unfriendly territory. I wanted to turn over all the trial and error triumphs and tragedies and help everyone. Experience after experience of people asking questions, pen in hand, taking down recommendations onto anything available to write on, prompted my writing down the top fifty suggestions, the essential things needed when headed into the cancer jungle. My wish is to touch every person facing cancer.

My dad, my hero, my daily encouragement and my protector, did not lose his battle to cancer. The doctors gave him 15 months and he lived 30 months. When I say he lived, he really lived: lived-it-up, lived every moment to the fullest, lived like tomorrow might never come, and went at life with everything he had. I have journals filled with the journeys, travels, laughter, jokes and love. I convinced myself day-in and day-out while the cancer process was in progress that the reason the tumor was found was to heal him and kill the cancer. Instead, it seems the reason was to offer us precious time together, after so many years where he and my mom worked so hard. I live in such gratitude now for that time, amongst the terror of cancer, as opposed to losing him suddenly.

Please keep in mind while reading that doctors go to medical school, nurses go to nursing school and I went to the school of spending two and a half years alongside a cancer patient in a hospital in gathering the recommendations outlined herein. I am not a doctor and no suggestions here are intended to diagnose, treat, cure, or prevent any disease. Moreover, the statements herein have not been evaluated by the Food and Drug Administration. You should always consult your own treating physician before beginning any protocol whatsoever, whether for diet, exercise, vitamins, over-the-counter medications, etc. In the case that your physician fails to help you in choosing an alternative medicine addition to your treatment, consider the help of a homeopathic physician.

This book was created solely from a first-hand learning process, motivated by the intense wish that my family would have gone into cancer knowing the hints offered in these pages. There is no association or endorsement intended between the author and any brand name, author, physician, or product mentioned in these pages. Any specific brand, author, physician or product mentioned herein resulted from personal experience with the product only. Every word here is designed to help and facilitate the cancer experience, not to treat or override the word of any physician, who is the only person who can say, for your type of diagnosis, treatment and body, what could be helpful or harmful.

This book resulted from the thirty months of painstaking learning. My intentions are to reach out a helping hand to the cancer patients, caregivers, families and friends facing this fight. I traveled to many of the top cancer treatment centers, moved across the country, gave up friends, family and familiarity to acquire the knowledge that I'd rather share than have learned in vain. I used to care about psychology, Broadway, movies and the newest books, now it sometimes seems that all I care about is cancer. I pray for the cures, seek understanding and continue a search for meaning and understanding through the aftermath of cancer.

I wish I could help every single patient and his or her family from the beginning to the end of their cancer journey. This book is my first step along that journey, while I discover where it takes me. My heart reaches out to each and every individual reading. I invite you to visit my website and email any thoughts or questions. I am willing to help in every way I can in any way I know how. You are not alone in this journey. Every cancer experience is as unique as the next. Keep always in the forefront of your mind that:

- ❖ Nearly every type of cancer at every stage has dissipated entirely, against all odds, and you could be another one of those patients.

- ❖ Apoptosis, the process of cancer cells committing suicide, occurs everyday throughout the world.

- ❖ The unknown and unexplainable still happens, everyday.

- ❖ It's perfectly reasonable to believe in miracles.

Chapter One ~ A Journey to Remember

Start a journal of the journey. Begin today. Include explanations, details, feelings, thoughts, facts, procedures, jokes, laughing moments, touching moments and even temper tantrums. Make them as long as pages a day or as short as a word or two. My specific cancer journalizing became very involved when the prognosis began looking severely grim as metastasis transpired. Now, four months of memories, laughs, cries, frustrating doctor appointments, moving moments, amongst more, fill several journals that warm and comfort me in my dad's physical absence, keeping specific memories alive.

Journaling the journey began the day I learned of the cancer diagnosis, however, it became lengthy and detailed, every single day, as things grew worse. Above all I strived to find one funny event that happened each day to record. I wrote about the little stories like the day I came home from shopping with my husband exhausted and asked my dad, "Is dinner ready?" as I knew he was working away at his famous pizza, that required twenty-four hours of preparation.

Shooting me an angry, exasperated look he answered, "We only have breadsticks and sauce."

"What? Why?" I replied.

Loudly, he barked back, "BECAUSE I DROPPED IT ON THE FLOOR, THAT'S WHY!"

"Oh, I'm sorry dad," I sheepishly said. His look of disappointment tugged at my heart. Chemotherapy consistently caused these glitches we weren't accustomed to that frustrated him terribly. I headed upstairs to call my husband for dinner. Returning back downstairs, a large pizza awaited on the stove. I sat staring at it with a confused expression. My dad burst into his uncontrollable, sidesplitting laughter. "You turkey!" I called out laughing.

"You should have seen your face!" he laughed. He was always such a jokester! When his health eventually began fading, the jokes became fewer and further between. I am eternally grateful I have pages and pages of his jokes and laughs to recall now.

The video camera always seems to lie dormant in its bag when the big moments happen. As much as we want to believe we will remember, memory fades. Moreover, the trauma from parts of the cancer experience sucks memory dry.

A journal provides a tangible legacy with the capacity of reminding oneself of both the horrendous and wondrous experiences later on. Regardless of the outcome of the cancer, the writings can serve as heirlooms and can be passed down later on. Also, the writings can document a life-changing journey. When recurrence occurred, for example, I discovered that one doctor, on a panel giving suggestions for treatment, recommended additional chemotherapy immediately following surgery. The other doctors recommended against chemotherapy. I felt incensed as we listened to the doctor explain when cancer reappeared, and considered the medical oncologist negligent, in retrospect. Then I pulled out a journal and read how my dad couldn't even walk downstairs in the house for such a long time after surgery, let alone have any quality of life. His medical oncologist felt, at the time, that more chemotherapy could kill him, and, reminding myself of reality by reading about the months after surgery, he was probably right. The reminder of days past quieted my rage.

Most my entries detail each day as specifically as the time restraints of any given day allowed. At other times, my strong feelings (not to mention exhaustion) led me to refrain from painting exactly how the day transpired and words like, "Chemo today. Sixteen hours at hospital" remain as the daily account. On other days, twenty pages or more remind me of moving details. On Halloween, as my journal recounts, Dad climbed in the passenger side of the Tahoe as we headed off for treatment. Tired already, I asked, "You got everything?"

"I shore do, girl," he answered in a thick redneck accent.

"DAD!" I shouted as I looked over at him smiling, ear-to-ear, with his fake, elaborate, costume teeth in. These yellow and brown stained teeth alternated with silver and gold teeth, the front top tooth displaying a star.

As we drove, he made eye-contact with others on the road, smiling at them, evoking both smiles and looks of horror among strangers. Walking into the hospital, he smiled at the receptionist, while wearing the teeth, calling out, "Howdy Mame." As we waited in the waiting room, he smiled around at unsuspecting patients and doctors alike. Some reacted with horror, others with laughs: he basked in every minute of the attention.

In the treatment room, he smiled and carried on in his thick hillbilly accent, with the teeth popping out crooked and with an extreme over-bite, he disgusted the nurse to the point that she stopped making eye-contact with him. "What's that there contraption you got?" he'd ask. Or when she asked him for his date of birth, he said, "Well, your a little early for my birthday, but only a few days, so I'll take the gift today if I got to." When she practically quit responding all together to him, dad popped the teeth out, put them in his pocket, and returned to his normal persona. The nurse re-entered the room and nearly fell over laughing.

"Oh my god, I'm so relieved," she said, laughing, "I really thought those were your teeth."

Dad got such a kick out of telling that story over and over!

My Dad missed his calling of being an actor. Thanks to my writing, though, my dad's gift lives on. Journaling, in any form, provides a wonderful suggestion for children, of any age, watching a loved one suffer through cancer. Pictures, words, stories, memories and experiences on paper act as great tools for self-expression and emotional health during this journey. My journals consisted of stories of how my dad made me laugh, moments together, wisdom he imparted, pictures of us in the hospital, out at dinner, or on vacation, in addition to the historical recounting of his treatment.

Paper accounts also provide a wonderful way of remembering doctor visit happenings, date history of the illness journey, and doctor inputs: all remarkable tracking devices that may prove valuable down the line. At more than one doctor's appointment, specific questions were asked regarding dates of treatment, side-effects experienced and other specifics not mentioned in medical charts that would have remained unanswered without my journals to reference. My dad said, after one doctor's appointment, "All that writing saves the day!"

The cancer patient, caregivers and family are all perfect candidates for journaling the cancer journey. Whatever the outcome of the cancer, you will be left with pages of priceless memories that will survive on, hopefully, in memory of the cancer battle triumphed over.

Chapter Two ~ Become Your Own Archivist

Initial diagnosis causes intense shock in combination with the flooding of thousands of other emotions. An intense desire to do something proactive often frustrates caregivers while waiting abounds as doctor visits are scheduled, therapies are set-up and the treatment ball begins rolling. As the process begins, get a three-ring binder as soon as possible. If the process has already begun, if half the treatment plan has passed, you can still begin with a binder today.

Collect copies of ALL laboratory work results this far, radiography reports, information given on specific drugs or protocols, doctor's cards and phone numbers for all important people to contact in each department, insurance information, advanced directives, and anything else gathered in the process. Buy plastic business card holders to put into the binder so all the doctor's cards can sit neatly arranged near the front of the binder for easy access. Or you can glue the cards onto a piece of paper and place it in the binder. Keep in mind that at the doctor's office cards should be gathered from the doctor, his or her nurse, his or her physician's assistant, his or her resident, his or her scheduler, etc. And thus five or six business cards may come from each doctor visited: the medical oncologist, radiation oncologist, surgical oncologist, pain management specialist, physical therapist, etc. Moreover, you may collect cards from patient advocates, hospital billing, pharmacies and other administrative offices involved in patient care.

With each laboratory visit, scan or new procedure, insist, before leaving the doctors office, you get a copy of the results. If you kindly ask a nurse, resident or doctor, the request should present no problem. Everyone involved in my father's care helpfully obliged the requests. Only records in bulk, like from six months or an entire year, seemed to create frustration and added work for hospital personnel and require anywhere from days to weeks to acquire.

Why are these papers important to keep? Isn't that the job of the doctor and/or hospital to keep track of all those? In some instances, doctors have failed to exam blood work closely enough. It takes no skill to read a report whatsoever. It consists of your result for the specific level, next to a normal range, where your number stands out in bold or has an asterisk beside it if the number lies out of the normal range. You need only examine your numbers against the normal ranges presented. Only knowledge of the progression of numbers, not a medical degree, is required to read lab reports. Results out of range often result in the adjustment of treatment. For instance, if a white blood cell count falls too low, doctors must postpone chemotherapy while presenting measures designed to increase the white blood cell count. A person who received chemotherapy after doctors overlooked a low white-cell count could face extreme illness or even death. Ask for a copy of blood work before every chemotherapy round. Become your own patient's advocate, double-checking a large, human system. Laboratory reports too often receive inadequate checking, or even go into a patient's file without anybody first reading them.

When my mother felt poorly at one time in her life, she received extensive blood work. The doctor reported all blood levels fell within normal limits, showing no obvious cause for her symptoms. Several months later, she felt worse, with frightening symptoms like severe chest pain, difficulty breathing, severe fatigue, acute weakness, among other symptoms. After running blood work again, this time at the emergency room, the treating physician discovered thyroid disease. Later in the week, after obtaining copies of the first blood work run, the reports displayed the presence of thyroid disease months ago, however the doctor had overlooked the number that lay clearly out of range. This same thing happened to our Golden Retriever and she almost died! We stopped relying solely on medical professionals to read reports far before cancer!

These laboratory reports prove critical to have on hand if need arises for a trip to the emergency room, especially if one lands in a position where need arises to rush to an emergency room at a different hospital than where he or she receives cancer treatment. In instances as these, one must also have on hand reports from any scans and the names of all drugs the person is receiving, in addition to the treating physicians' contact information. This will dramatically improve the quality and promptness of treatment.

Additionally, if the need arises for a second opinion at a hospital in the next city over, or, more drastically, if you decide to move three thousand miles to a different cancer hospital, you will need all afore mentioned paperwork. Collecting it piece-by-piece, at each appointment, and placing it in a binder will greatly help in the case that you leave your hospital for any reason. To get all the reports and information copied from the hospital we left when recurrence arose would have required weeks of notice. These institutions busily treat hundreds to thousands of patients, and most cannot stop on a dime to collect and copy an individual's records even within that same week. Instead you must be patient. Patience proves nearly impossible with a looming cancer diagnosis or news of recurrence.

In our case we had no idea we were moving to Houston. One day we were flying to Houston to vacation and have a check-up with the surgeon who had moved from Los Angeles to Houston, literally, the next week we were moved to Houston. There would have been little time or patience to stop and collect all records. There was no need; they were already in two large three-ring binders. As a result we saw the medical oncologist on a Thursday and received chemotherapy on Friday: an amazing payoff for gathering one or two pieces of paper each time we left a doctors appointment. I figure, for the amount I pay to see the doctor, I want to leave with something tangible in my hand! They at least owe me a piece of paper!

My hope is that one day in the near future, all patients will receive the results from their tests and other crucial paperwork at every doctor appointment as a required part of the visit. The bill for those blood tests comes to my house, not the doctors, so I expect to see what I paid for. Moreover, I hope we all begin keeping medical binders to take back some power over our own health care.

Cancer treatment is not predictable, simplistic or straightforward. Increase your chances of having the best treatment possible by collecting and keeping your own records. Check with your doctor. Become an active part of your own care. Prepare for the worst so you free yourself up to hope for the best.

Chapter Three ~ Scrap Book the Mementos

Create memories and turn them into memory albums. Scrap booking is spreading like wildfire as we move from albums containing only pictures to albums with pictures, ticket stubs, stickers, and memories written beside pictures among other memorabilia. Cancer, we decided, would create memories whether we wanted it to or not. Using creativity and experiences, we packed books full of memorabilia from pictures at chemo, hospital bracelets, pictures arriving home from the hospital, amongst trips we made in between ranging from birthdays to vacations. The memories, we figured, would be priceless either way: either memories of a triumphant journey; or priceless treasures from our last adventures. Our books created throughout cancer turned out to be both. Eventually, they will be both for everyone.

My dad participated in making pages with us, leaving us with the memories in the pictures and in the creation of the scrapbooks as well. My sister's eighteenth birthday arrived a few months after my dad's surgery. As a gift we created an elaborate scrapbook album for her, my dad taking time to choose pictures and then write his memories, thoughts and birthday wishes. For instance, beside the pictures of the car she got for her sixteenth birthday that dad wrapped in a big red ribbon were his memories written, on a large cut-out of a stop sign, of her driving test. What a priceless gift to have now, with his writing and love, always easily accessible in that album. Pictures of my dad in the first rounds of chemo, where he had to stay for inpatient therapy, reminded us of the beginning. We remember taking him home on his birthday when we brought balloons, party hats and presents to his discharge. We remember bringing him home from surgery on Valentine's Day and have pictures out front of our home where we had decorated the house and his truck: he was so happy to be home! Our scrapbooks are packed to the brim: we included trips to Memphis, Nashville, Orlando, Branson, Austin, Louisiana, Oklahoma, Arkansas, Mississippi, Houston, San Antonio and Dallas alongside walks around the bayou next to our home and fun times at home. Pictures in Dallas remind us of the adventure we took to flee Hurricane Rita in the midst of cancer treatment.

My dad suffered with pain and exhaustion at that point and grew extremely agitated in the massive exodus from the city that turned a 250-mile drive into a twelve-hour excruciating journey. Next to a picture of the hotel where we ended up, I recount a story of being in the elevator with my irritable dad. We had our Golden Retriever with us who has one eye, after a tumor claimed the other eye. Three intoxicated guys wandered into the elevator and asked what happened to her eye. We were all tired and worn out, not in the mood to tell the story, so my dad spoke up and explained, "Well, she saved a cub scout who was being attacked by a bear. She fought that bear with all her might. But she lost her eye. It was the price she had to pay for saving that boy's life." The guys bought the story hook, line and sinker. The mood instantaneously turned from irritability to sidesplitting laughter.

Certain brands of scrapbook materials are unique in that they enable a person to order supplies and have them delivered. Delivery proves especially simple in the midst of cancer. The best brands to choose promote photo-safe products that help ensure photos and memories will last many lifetimes. Scrap booking stores abound to offer classes, ideas, stickers, papers, scissors, stamps, and overwhelming creativity. Online scrap booking sites will let you find stickers and scrap booking materials for practically anything.

Many arts and crafts stores now also offer extensive scrap booking sections. Tourist attractions often carry their own exclusive line of products to help add to the creation of memories from special trips. In buying scrap-booking products from tourist attractions, keep in mind that if you purchase the book and its pages at the location, ensure you have enough pages to complete the book. If you do not purchase enough pages at the time, you may run into problems. For instance, in Disneyworld, we strayed from our typical scrap-booking brand and purchased a beautiful, unique scrapbook. Back home, creating the album, we discovered we needed 20 or 30 more pages to complete the album. We searched site after site and store after store, but could not find the correct page covers anywhere. It required a pricey and creative solution that we made work, but could have been prevented by purchasing enough pages in Disneyworld when we were there.

My scrapbooks are my most cherished keepsakes now in the aftermath of cancer: the sweetest tangible gift my dad left behind! Cancer will make memories and impact our lives. With scrap booking, one can embrace time together while ensuring the memory lives on. Scrap booking can leave the family with a positive product from cancer, regardless of the outcome of cancer itself.

Chapter Four ~ Vitamin Power

Vitamins played a crucial role in our health as a family through cancer. My dad had a month-and-a-half waiting period before treatment could begin. Vitamins and dietary supplements bestowed some peace of mind that perhaps we were doing something to help during the waiting period. If nothing else, perhaps, through adding health we were strengthening his immune system and body for the fight ahead.

Obviously this presents neither scientific study nor proof, but through countless different chemotherapy drugs (two treatments so potent that he had to remain hospitalized throughout the treatment as he received intravenous chemotherapy for twenty-four hours a day, for seven days straight), radiation, two surgeries, biological therapy and clinical trials, aside from cancer, my dad retained his health, never contracting any cold, cough, flu, etc. This proves rather remarkable and extraordinary when considering the immune system undergoes intentional destruction when undergoing chemotherapy and he visited the hospital daily for sixty days, stayed in the hospital for weeks and went out and about around people, where germs abound.

As caregivers, my mom, sister and I also took high-quality, natural vitamins daily. In previous years we typically caught several colds a year: sinus infections, bronchitis, strep throat, etc. When cancer began, we all sought the assistance of vitamins in remaining healthy. That year, even in the face of the stress of cancer, we remained much healthier than usual. This proves vital, not only for self-care for the caregiver, but also for the patient as well, seeing that sick people in the house present a direct, and often serious threat to the patient undergoing cancer treatment.

My dad never spent a night wearing a facemask, gloves or other germ protecting devises and yet he remained remarkably healthy. Though my family popped grocery store brand vitamins for years, we strongly believe our switch to high-quality, all-natural vitamins made a difference. At times it seemed a nuisance that the particular brand we chose could, almost exclusively, only be purchased online or by ordering through a representative, however, the delivery proves extremely convenient through cancer. Above all, I recommend investigating the sources involved in the creation of any vitamin taken. I found the high-quality, naturally derived vitamins, from a variety of brands, help contribute to health and immune strength.

There are different philosophies and views on vitamins through cancer treatment. In my father's case, the best oncologist for his type of cancer found a multi-vitamin harmless and recommended it. Other doctors feel differently. During treatment, doctor's recommendations should be followed about all else. Also keep in mind that treatments, depending on the type and dosage, remain in the system for several weeks.

Caregivers also should consult their general practitioner and call on vitamins to help maintain health during cancer. They help energy, boost the immune system and prevent illness while you care for the ill. Dr. Forrest C. Shaklee created one of the first multivitamins in 1915. Since vitamins have undergone many changes. I continue to choose Shaklee, as it is important to me to select a vitamin containing the most natural ingredients, those that harm neither the person nor the environment. I also ensure the vitamin products I purchase are not tested on animals, are free of preservatives, artificial sweeteners, colors, flavors, or any other artificial ingredients.

Experiment with a trial period: keep track of energy, mood, health and overall well being while adding a vitamin regimen. Consult your physician and investigate the natural vitamin options available to you. Any assistance in the fight against cancer is worth a shot.

Chapter Five ~ Support Lance Armstrong

Visit Lance Armstrong's website. The resources, materials and support available at the website prove amazing. Spend time gaining from Armstrong's experience and effort: his books, his bracelet's, and his cancer binder. He's truly an American hero! Walking around with a yellow band around your wrist reminds you of all those united together in this cancer battle together.

Chapter Six ~ Investigate Your Insurance Website

Health insurance companies have websites that hold a wealth of tools and information readily available for you. Extensive time lapsed before I found this invaluable tool, as before cancer I had little need for the landscape of information available at my insurance website. My favorites on my insurance website consist of the pharmacy tools and wellness tips. Many insurance sites also have registered nurses available for consultation twenty-four hours a day! The insurance site proved indispensable to the point of getting a portable, internet-ready device I could take to the hospital. The reason for the necessity was the result of the following true story.

Pain management proved a growing challenge. As my father waited until the pain grew to a rather serious level before taking pain medication, it became necessary to have a fast-acting pain solution. Severe acute pain set in while waiting to see a doctor, sending us scurrying over to the pain management specialist. She quickly handed him oral transmucosal fentanyl citrate, the pain pop, as they called it. Rubbing the sucker-like stick containing fentanyl on the inside of the cheek and gums delivers rather prompt, short-acting pain relief, allowing time for long-lasting pain medication to work. The pain pop saved the day, and the doctor quickly wrote out a prescription.

We delivered the prescription to the hospital pharmacy so it could be filled before we left. As afternoon fell on a Friday, we figured it would be quite late before we returned home and so we turned the prescription into the hospital pharmacy. The pharmacy said, "Our pharmacy doesn't accept your insurance, if we fill it, it will cost

$1500. You should take it somewhere your insurance covers."

It struck us as odd: 'The hospital takes our insurance, but their pharmacy doesn't?' we thought. No need to argue; who wants to pay $1500 for something insurance covers? Arriving home at about nine that evening, we drove through the pharmacy drop-off. They asked us to return for pick-up in two-and-a-half hours. Considering the necessity of the medication, we decided we would return. Resorting to pots of coffee to stay awake, we struggled to keep our eyes open after a long day at the hospital. At 11:30 pm, at the pharmacy window, the pharmacist explained, "You need prior authorization on this. Since it's Friday night, we won't be able to call the doctor until Monday. We should be able to get it to you by Wednesday." Nobody seems to care you have a suffering cancer patient at home when a policy dictates something that conflicts with what you need.

Although I still do not understand the issue of prior authorization after a cancer diagnosis, I know I ran into three medications in the course of cancer requiring prior authorization. Prior authorization proves non-problematic only if you ensure the doctor calls your insurance and gives prior authorization before 5pm on any day of the week. This becomes a nightmare after 5 o'clock on any Friday.

Our systems, advanced as they have become, remain computers rather than humans. When the pharmacy says, "You need prior authorization. Your insurance only covers this for cancer," you can only shake your head over the nonsensical part of that. I explained, "The prescription is from a cancer center and the insurance obviously knows by now he has cancer." It simply does not work that way. I learned quickly to run a pharmacy check on the insurance website before leaving the doctor's office. If prior authorization was necessary, I could then inform the doctor and have him or her call the insurance company and pharmacy before we left. On the insurance website I can see how many pills, patches, suckers, etc. are allowed, if prior authorization is required and if there are restrictions. On one anti-nausea medication, the doctor could over-ride the insurance's restriction of only nine pills allowed at a time, keeping us from running to the pharmacy every other day.

The word "prior" in prior authorization actually means prior to 5pm, especially on Friday's. Nobody ever mentioned prior authorization to me, nor had I ever experienced it after years of going to the pharmacy. The worst time to learn is in the midst of is suffering. Find a way to quickly check prior authorizations. Maybe there is a pharmacy line for your insurance you can call, maybe you will invest in a cellular phone with internet capabilities, perhaps the hospital has a computer center, conceivably you could call someone with access to the internet and have them check the insurance website. Finding someway to prevent learning a prior authorization is needed at 5pm will make life easier!

Chapter Seven ~ The Very Special Specialist

Pain management proves a vital part of cancer care and treatment. Everything from a tumor itself to surgery, chemotherapy, radiation and metastasis can induce incredible pain. Contrary to what many people believe from the old days of cancer treatment, many drugs at many dosages now exist to treat your type and degree of pain. Many think of pain management in cancer as limited to morphine. As pain management has risen to its own specialty in itself, cancer patients now hold an abundance of options.

Pain management specifically for cancer patients is breaking out as a rather new phenomenon available at the top cancer centers in the country. There, I learned, they have "tricks" to treat the pain that the oncologists, clinical trials team or palliative care do not even know about. Just as the oncologist presents the newest chemo drugs and the surgeon studies advances in surgical procedure, the pain management specialist knows about the newest pain medications on the market and how they stop the, often invasive, pain of cancer.

While some, unaccustomed to the highly specialized method of medicine sweeping our country, find the pain management specialist superfluous when their other entourage of doctors can treat the pain, many of the top doctors in the country are now insisting that procuring a pain management specialist is crucial in receiving top care. To the pain management opponents, I ask, would you allow your medical oncologist to operate on you? The obvious response follows, "Not in this highly specialized day and age."

Even at one of the top cancer centers in the country we found the oncologist, the oncologist's assistant, the oncologist's resident, the oncologist's nurse, the team of doctors in palliative care, the doctors in radiation oncology and then the doctors in clinical trials, insisting their pain medications and their pain management was just as good as the pain management team; that their treatments would follow the same protocol as their pain management specialist peers. Please hear this: they were not the same treatments, they did not follow the same protocols, and the pain management specialists were the only team that completely stopped the pain! In the highly specialized world of medicine, each physician comprising the treatment team has received highly specialized education and continued education in cancer treatment. The pain management specialist primarily studies pain treatment options. Pain degrades the life of the suffering cancer patient to the point that having a pain management specialist would be a higher priority in my treatment team than many other specialists.

How does pain management differ between the other doctors and the pain management specialist? The pain management specialist treats pain in its entirety. As the pain progressed we had a sustained-release pain medication, a breakthrough pain medication, a short-term breakthrough pain medication to alleviate pain until the other medications began working, in addition to daily pain medication. The "pain pop" or the cancer medication in sucker form for short-term breakthrough pain was unknown to the oncologists' staff, radiation oncologist's staff, the clinical trials staff, the emergency room staff and hospital staff in a cancer treatment hospital! That offered demonstration enough that our pain management team remained essential. Moreover, cancer pain management specialists also carry non-drug tools to use alone (if the patient wishes) or in conjunction with drug therapies.

One aspect of pain management in cancer treatment that causes concern is addiction. Addiction concerns arose in our home. But time and time again, top oncologists explained in detail that pain addiction among cancer patients is incredibly low. Moreover, some of the unfortunate side effects of pain medication also arise in patients experiencing pain not taking pain medication. Oncologists from all walks agree the effects of pain on the body are worse than the consequences of many pain medications. Consider this fact alone: the body's most powerful weapon against cancer, the immune system, is suppressed by pain. Pain is an enemy in the fight against cancer.

Another myth involved in pain management involves the belief that doctors will over-medicate cancer patients, leaving them feeling "doped up" all the time. This idea reflects old-school cancer pain treatments that pain specialist's work diligently to correct. And if you do find yourself over-medicated: tell somebody or find another doctor, because it is not necessary. At one time our clinical trial team attempted to up my father's medication from hydromorphone to methadone. The pain management specialist interceded, stepping the medication up gradually, stopping pain, while preventing the dopey feeling.

A pain management specialist can also be a powerful ally prior to hospice, if hospice becomes necessary. When hospice entered our lives, we argued only that the working pain treatment regimen remain as it was or we would call in another hospice company. Hospice is a big business, just as any other medical treatment, and you should have a voice in your treatments, even with hospice on scene. If hospice fails in completely managing your pain, you can withdraw from hospice, visit a cancer pain management specialist, and then re-join hospice (as most insurance companies will not pay for doctor visits while a patient is under hospice treatment.)

The most significant reason for having a pain management specialist is that it gives you a doctor around the clock, everyday of the year, responsible for nothing but freeing you from pain so your body can focus on fighting cancer. "How long do I wait for pain to subside?" I once asked a prominent oncologist.

"Within 24 hours of trying and not receiving the desired relief, start calling the pain doctor," he answered. "There is no reason, with the advanced pain medications we now have, for physical suffering. If there's physical suffering longer than that, it's your fault for not getting pain management on the line." Cancer is stressful, exhausting, consuming, confusing, worrisome, bothersome and many other things; it should not be painful too. Cancer pain specialists present a powerful tool not yet fully utilized in cancer pain treatment. If you have physical pain as a result of your cancer, find a cancer pain management specialist today!

Chapter Eight ~ Rally Support

Support from friends and family during cancer is so needed that a surplus seems impossible. Never do you sit in a cancer treatment hospital or the oncologist's office hearing, "If only I had less support, this battle would be easier." And yet, despite our newspapers, magazines, television and internet abounding with the discussion of cancer, albeit 1.4 million new diagnoses each year, still people run from cancer like it's the plague. Not knowing what to say, unsure of what to do, unsure if you want to talk about it, hoping to avoid upsetting you, avoiding making you feel uncomfortable, people often fall silent, creating distance that leaves a patient feeling upset, uncared for and uncomfortable. Some of the worst people we dealt with were even family and friends, some who had gone through cancer themselves!

To help my dad feel supported and loved, I employed a highly recommended mode of support. I obtained a prayer pager for my dad, and then sent the number out to hundreds of people, asking them to send their prayers, thoughts and well wishes anytime they had a spare minute. Finding a pager created more of a hurdle than I imagined, but it allowed people to know they could leave messages rather than face an actual discussion about cancer. This allows a way for the cancer patient to feel cared about while also giving family and friends a specific way to care. Every month or so I would send an update, explaining, "So now he's going in to another inpatient round of treatment," or "Surgery is only a week away," so people could receive reminders that support still helped!

The idea has many variations. Websites can be put up to ask people to post messages, text messages can be requested, and email allows a number of possibilities. Putting up a website with a schedule, needed help and other information can help create a thriving support network. Posting a "help-needed" section can give people who want to offer a helping hand specific ways to help. It might read, "Lawn mowed, dog walked, dry cleaning picked up, someone to sit with him/her for an hour on Tuesday."

People, in general, really want to help and support, but have no idea how. To be totally honest, the person who gave the most support and care during cancer came for a visit and asked to take my dad for a small walk. After my dad died, the person exclaimed, "If I'd have known how bad it was, I would have done more." What I explained was my dad talked about that gesture of kindness and support frequently. As odd as it may sound to a person or family facing cancer, asking for support and giving specifics will help keep support around at such a tumultuous time in life.

Chapter Nine ~ Pharmacy Patient Etiquette

Imagine the following scenario: On a Friday evening you pull out of the parking structure after a twelve-hour day at the medical center. Celebrating a twelve-hour day (last time entailed a sixteen hour hospital day), you dream of your bed. Your loved one sleeps in the passenger seat: cancer is exhausting. After dropping the pain medication prescription off at the twenty-four-hour pharmacy and stopping quickly by home to let your loved one crawl into bed, you return to the pharmacy for the prescription. But, it falls on a Friday during flu season, so the pharmacist apologizes, it will take four hours. Too tired to try another pharmacy, you decide to return in four hours, even though that will mean a midnight run to the pharmacy.

It takes an entire pot of coffee, but you're still up and finally 11:30 pm rounds. At 11:45 pm the pharmacist says, "You're prescription won't be ready until midnight." So you walk around the store, afraid that if you sit down, you'll fall asleep right there in the pharmacy. Finally, both hands line up along the twelve and you crawl to the counter. You give your name. The pharmacist walks away, returning empty-handed. "We don't have this medication. You'll have to wait until at least Tuesday, maybe Wednesday." Not only do you not have the medication that you know will be needed come six am, you now also have to deal with a ridiculous drama of having the prescription removed from the "system" that they insist it cannot be taken out of, and you also have to go on a search to find a pharmacy that is a) open and b) has the drug, while you try to keep yourself from decking the pharmacist.

One first hand experience with this story proves one too many. For us, in some variation or another, it occurred time and time again until finally we learned to ask, EVERY SINGLE TIME, upon dropping off any prescription, "Could you please check to make sure you have the drug before I leave?" And make sure they have the brand name if you want it, because sometimes a pharmacist's "Yes" means, "Yes, we have some variation of that drug." So my conversations went as follows, every single time:

"Here's my prescription and could you please check to see if you have that before I go?"

The pharmacist would return. "Yes, we have it in stock."

"So, you have (x) number of (y) drug?" I would follow up to ensure I would receive a full fill (rather than a partial fill) of the drug I wanted (and not a substitute, if I didn't want a substitute.)

And it seems every time I forgot to go through this conversation, I ended up with some version of the above story. The time the pharmacist said she didn't have time to check, I began my most dramatic version of the above story, which you might want to memorize and perform as your own incase they say they don't have time. She made time after that story. Take my suffering and use it to prevent your own. For some reason with pharmacies and cancer, Murphy's Law was the rule of thumb.

Chapter Ten ~ The Vomit Vessel

Nausea and vomiting are difficult aspects of cancer and cancer treatment. Everyone involved finds it unpleasant and stressful. Try as we might with nausea remedies, nausea and vomiting will most likely will occur at some point. To simplify life and ease a patient's mind, purchase or designate some vomiting receptacle, and place it near wherever the patient spends the majority of his or her down time. For us, it was a large yellow plastic bowl that had seen a fruit salad too many. Inexpensive suitable options abound in neighborhood superstores or even grocery stores. Other ideas are small plastic wastebaskets, buckets left over from laundry detergent or specified bowls at medical supply stores. In my case, feeling the most "normal" and least "medical" made a large bowl most ideal. Multiple receptacles may create convenience, depending on the severity of the nausea, with one beside the bed, one beside the couch, one in the car, etc.

Cancer patients can feel tired, weak and completely out-of-it. A vomit bowl can allow the patient to remain in place. Moreover, it allows one to exert less energy than running to the bathroom. Also, it gives ease of mind that if nausea or vomiting creep up on a person, the bowl or receptacle waits nearby. Finally, spending time bent over a toilet, lying on a bathroom floor or lounging in the bathroom with a lingering feeling of nausea presents increased risk to an individual's health. The bathroom abounds with germs: it's simply not where a cancer patient needs to lounge around, or spend more time than is necessary. Studies show toothbrushes left on the sink can have remnants of fecal material on them from being spewed out of the toilet during flushing, so imagine what one could acquire while lying on the floor!

Vomit is one of the rougher parts of cancer. It just seems wrong that an illness and treatments that inflict such fatigue and weakness should be allowed to have vomiting as a side effect. Using love and care for a cancer patient by overcoming negative reactions and helping in a loving, yet noninvasive manner, helps. For my dad it was providing the bowl, handing over wet towels and wet paper towels, stepping out of view, but keeping close enough to return if needed, and then empting the bowl and rubbing his back. But beyond anything we could do as caregivers, that bowl was a lifesaver!

Chapter Eleven ~ Obtain a Moss Report

"What else can I do to help?"

"What if the doctor says there's no hope?"

"Is this alternative treatment available for this type of cancer worth a grain of salt?"

"What does the newest research say?"

"Where do I find answers pertaining to my type of cancer?"

"Which alternative treatments are mainly just about profiting from cancer?"

You can find the answers to these questions with one quick stop. Check out Ralph Moss' website and sign up for free weekly newsletters. Ralph Moss has conducted independent research for thirty plus years, evaluating various cancer treatments in both conventional and alternative realms. He has written consistently updated reports regarding specifics on over two hundred different types of cancer. The reports consist of several hundred pages each! In each report he discusses the best Western medical approaches to each specific type of cancer, in addition to alternative medical approaches, unbiased and scientifically lending credit to both sides. He neither rallies for the western medical approach nor alternative medicine; rather he relies on evidence and research and reports his findings.

His weekly reports offer fascinating, cutting-edge cancer research in user friendly, readable reports. Does sunscreen cause skin cancer or prevent skin cancer? Is açai a hope or a hoax? Are radio frequency energy fields causing cancer? He studies the newest medical and alternative treatments alike, evaluating the biased views on each side. In the field of cancer, gallant human beings striving for cures in conventional and alternative medicine work tirelessly. Unfortunately, some also focus on profit and promoting their products. Regardless of each sides motivations and intentions, each frequently discredit the other, leaving consumers confused. Ralph Moss stands in the middle to call on the data (including both scientific and case studies) to sort through discrepancies between contradicting views on cancer topics.

Now, the Moss Reports offer you support and evaluations in mere moments, as they come in electronic format. They remain available via standard mail delivery as well. Check out Ralph Moss' biography, and explore the resources on his website. Beyond the report, he and his staff are available for phone consultations. First, however, they expect you to thoroughly read the report on your type of cancer, to avoid having to repeat the resources they have already compiled in the reports.

The Moss Reports became like a cancer bible along our journey. The cost proves cheap when considering the wealth of information they offer. My dad's cancer never received an absolute diagnosis of where it originated. Some called it esophageal cancer that traveled south, others called it gastric cancer that stretched north, while still there were those who referred to it as cancer of the gastro-esophageal junction. Thus, after receiving the Moss Report on gastric adenocarcinoma, we also ordered the esophageal cancer and gastro-esophageal junction cancer Moss Reports as well.

Examine Moss' books while at his website as well: they extend practical help and hope, offering fantastic cancer support. His books provide more affordable overviews, whereas the specific reports give the complete analysis for very specific types of cancer.

Visit www.ralphmoss.com today.

Chapter Twelve ~ All Hours Support Lifeline

Cancer, as my stories might illustrate, took a deep and serious toll on my entire life. My spirit, my heart, my health, my emotional state and my psyche all suffered. In my position, going to support groups, while they were absolutely fantastic, required more energy than remained at the end of most care-giving days. Without the groups, I began feeling lost and alone. Nobody understood the pain, anguish and exhaustion. Every time I went out: the grocery store, the post office, the pharmacy, restaurants, the hardware store, etc., I felt more alienated and more alone in cancer.

Then, I stumbled upon online support groups. There was one for the specific type of cancer, patients only, caregivers, alternative treatments, conventional treatments, new breakthrough drugs, etc. And I joined them all. Each group pulled a massive thorn from my side. These online support groups allowed a quick and easy, nearly always accessible, group of friends, comrades in battle. When I read stories of the same stressors, frustrations and breakdowns as I experienced, I felt so much more normal and less alone. When I read about people who lost loved ones, I felt appreciation for the time I still had. When I read about situations far worse than my own, I felt grateful for what I did have. When I felt my situation was unbearable, I could share my thoughts and feelings and receive an outpouring of support from others in similar situations.

Check out the popular search engine communities for their group sections. Once you find the group section, search for the part of the cancer experience that you are looking for: cancer patients, your specific type of cancer, caregivers, children of parents with cancer, etc. Specific sites also exist to direct you to online support. "Cancer Care" and "The Wellness Community" both have sites to help search for support groups for your type of cancer, caregiving, treatments and more.

Online support groups provide a place to ask, "Has anybody else experienced this side effect from this drug?" "Does anyone have any suggestions for what I can do to help this problem?" "Are there specific questions I can ask the doctor about this problem?" among a thousand other questions. Upon joining, active participation is not a requirement. Reading all the posts from other members offers help and support as well. Witnessing others' feelings of isolation and frustration, hearing of other individuals with hopeful stories, learning about a new anti-nausea medication, and finding a beneficial website can strongly impact your journey through cancer as a patient, caregiver or family member.

Proximity to medical centers, longs lists of chores, wanting to spend quality time in the face of cancer, inability to leave without many preparations and pure exhaustion made physical attendance at support groups nearly impossible for me to incorporate on a regular basis. But the online support groups saved me. When my dad contracted a case of hiccups that lasted days on end, a recommendation from someone on a caregivers group helped me request a medication to stop the hiccups. Bizarre side effects from one treatment caused great alarm, but others on a support group for the new drug confirmed they had traveled that road as well, and helped give many suggestions to ease the pain associated with the side effects. Sorrow and grief that arose when metastasis spread drove many to offer books, websites and suggestions to support and comfort during dark times.

By all means go to support groups at your hospital, medical center, church or community center. I strongly suggest supplementing those support groups with virtual support groups as well. The around the clock support, right there in your home (or in the hospital via internet on your cell phone), will keep hundreds of others busy fighting the same battle at an arms reach, ready to help and encourage.

Chapter Thirteen ~ Inspect Pharmacy Bottles

Check your pill bottles from the pharmacy *carefully*. Check the name on the bottle (not just the outside of the bag). Make sure that it is YOUR name. If you have a common name, check additional information on the label, like your address. Then, after you have ensured they have your information correct, check your doctor's information.

After moving to a different cancer center, we were subjected to pharmacies where we faced one problem after another. Consistently the doctor's name was incorrect on the label. At first, in the midst of the exhaustion of cancer, we let it go, thinking, 'what does it really matter? Not like it's affecting the medication.' Then, one day the pharmacy called the doctor for authorization to refill the prescription. We arrived to pick-up the medication and learned the doctor had denied the refill. Much valuable time slipped by figuring out why the doctor rejected the refill. Finally, we learned "the doctor" rejected the refill, claiming he did not have a patient by that name. As a result of the pharmacy putting the wrong doctor on the bottle, we then were required to return to the hospital for another paper prescription. As it turns out, the doctor's name being correct on your label IS important!

Once verifying the information on the label, consider counting the pills. Pay special attention if dealing with pain medication, sleeping medication and chemotherapy drugs. The black market for pills of this nature makes the pills highly valuable to some people. Depending on the type of medication, some of these pills sell on the street for ten to fifty dollars a pill! Whether my luck was based on sticky fingers or something else, I cannot say, but my experience was always receiving bottles of these prescriptions with one to three pills missing, especially with pain medications. Whether a coincidence or not, my "boring" prescriptions were always correct!

I initially felt crazy sitting in the drive-thru counting pills. Quickly I learned the joke was on me if I did not count! Do keep in mind some medications should not be touched at all or by people other than the patient. Regardless of whether you want to take it as far as I do with the counting, check for absolute accuracy of the label. Be sure to have the prescribing doctor's full name, address and phone number on hand when filling prescriptions. Believe it or not, we experienced several doctors who were not in the pharmacy's system, which required us giving the physician's phone number and address for the medication to receive proper labeling. I joke that cancer made my family my dad's advocates, nurses, doctors and pharmacists!

Chapter Fourteen ~ The Book for Life

Life Lessons, a book by Elisabeth Kübler-Ross and David Kessler, became a daily reading for me during cancer. While I fretted endlessly over if this treatment would work, would he feel better, would things get better, would he die, how much time did he have left and what else could we do, Life Lessons showed me how to transcend my fear, terror and stress, how to enjoy moments, and how to truly live in the face of cancer.

Life Lessons, a collaboration of Elisabeth Kübler-Ross and David Kessler, arrived after spending countless hours with the dying, offering the crucial points for really living. When my dad reached a point where he knew the end was coming, when he could only receive food, water and medicine by a feeding tube and could not even swallow water, he knew more about life than he ever did. He said, "Live every day. Appreciate the ability to get up and do things." Tears slid down his face, as he longed to get up, and he offered, "Don't take your health and body for granted." He said, "Don't worry so much." In a quiet, peaceful simplicity he shared, "I spent too much time being angry." I understood. He was saying all my anger was useless. In listening to his wisdom, I understand why wisdom, depth and simple suggestions for living, especially in the face of something like cancer, spill from every page of Life Lessons. Elisabeth Kübler-Ross, known for all her work on death, truly perfected living and, with David Kessler, they gifted the world with presenting the keys to life through Life Lessons.

I am a huge fan of all Elisabeth Kübler-Ross' and David Kessler's books. Search both authors and see if their titles or collaborations interest you. When my dad began dying, Elisabeth Kübler-Ross' On Death and Dying helped me tremendously with my psychological and mental pain of impending death. David Kessler's The Needs of the Dying helped perfectly with understanding the physical process of death and approaching needs. In the aftermath of cancer, their collaboration On Grief and Greiving helps me more than any other single book for my grief and heartache after death.

Read Life Lessons. It truly gives peace in the face of cancer. I have read most cancer books, most books in the Self-Help section and a great deal of psychology books, and yet I find Life Lessons continuously remains number one on my list. It belongs in a section all of its own in the bookstore. It's the book I take everywhere, the one I would choose if I could only read one book for the rest of my life. As Elisabeth Kübler-Ross' last book, she and Mr. Kessler left the world with one glistening magnificent treasure.

Chapter Fifteen ~ Make Movies

During cancer, video can become one more stressful thing that nobody has the energy to do. I know because somehow my videoing-obsessed family, moved by exhaustion and desire to live in the moment, videoed less than ever. Now, in the face of loss after cancer that we neither expected nor truly fathomed, we cherish the moments on video we have and wish that while we were living "in the here and now" we would have had the video on more. We would have turned it on and left it on a tripod during dinner, while we cooked and watched the parade on Thanksgiving, while we watched a movie together or played cards on some idle Wednesday night. The video would have been on, even if only paid minor attention to, while we were in Disneyworld, at the Grand Ole Opry, or on travels through the great state of Texas. In videoing, even with minor attention focused on the shot, I would have more moments of my dad's voice, the music of his laughter and the spark that his smile ignited.

Videoing is never wasted. Whatever the unknown outcome of cancer, memories stored on tape can serve as a memory of the cancer process you made it through, a great gift to pass down and will make for great enjoyment if at 90 you can watch it and reminisce what you all lived through! It's a win-win situation.

One video treasure I can share came from a trip to Disneyworld, in the midst of cancer and cancer treatment. I brought along the video one night and propped it up to record, practically hanging it on the end of my hand, at the table. My dad, the clown, turned into an absolute entertainment act at a French restaurant in Disneyworld. I captured it all on film! He begins with reading the French menu in a midwestern accent. He then recites French phrases he knew from a specific French learning method, where memorization of phrases abounds, insisting he was going to repeat them to the waiter, like "Où est-ce que vous habitez, Jacques?" (where do you live, Jack?). He ordered soup, then began eating it with his mouth inches from the bowl, slurping each spoonful like a child. After, he began dancing to Japanese drumming, and was so entertaining even passing strangers laughed. After arriving home, we found the video hilarious. Now, without his frequent live entertainment, the video is priceless.

Another idea for cancer patients is making videos for loved ones, now while you can, to have to leave behind in case death approaches. I know of many parents who videoed for their children, ensuring their presence during major life milestones, regardless of the outcome of cancer. My dad went from believing he had decades to live to days to live so fast that by the time I asked him to make a video or write a card for my sisters 21st birthday, he said "I'm sorry, I can't." I held absolute optimism, hope and belief in a cure. If my Dad would have made videos or something of that nature, I would have been upset at the time, but now I wish I had a video message directed to me more than anything in the world. I would watch it every day. It would be the best gift. I know because the videos I have are monumental gifts.

A final idea concerning videos involves video slideshows. Fantastic as birthday or Christmas gifts, or perhaps just as a celebration of life, slideshows with photographs, video clips, captions and music can be created. The website I found which will put as many photographs as you choose, the music you choose, video clips and captions if you wish, and turn it into a wonderful slideshow with fantastic effects, www.permanenttreasures.com, will create an amazing gift for you and your family to share for generations to come. After my dad passed, the mortuary made a slideshow. It was a nightmare. The pictures were blurry, we could not have music of our choice, there were no effects and it was extremely expensive. Permanent Treasures met all my needs, allowed me to preview my slideshow to make changes and had moving effects. Their slideshows are works of art!

Capture moments and memories on video. Cancer creates intense fear about tomorrow, but videoing is about preserving memories and creating treasures. Videoing, video memorials and slideshows celebrate today, celebrate life and celebrate love. Cancer, inevitably at times, creates fear, heartache, pain, worry and a thousand other negative emotions; but through making memories the negative emotions associated with cancer fade into the background while the life available today moves into the spotlight.

Chapter Sixteen ~ Pill Row

Pillboxes become as precious as treasure chests when facing the pill regimen cancer often entails. In my own experience, pillboxes did not come into play or become helpful until pain medications entered the mix. Unfortunately, it skipped our minds that pillboxes would greatly help. Forgetting about pillboxes, we first had to experience toting around pain medication bottles from the pharmacy with us to the hospital, the grocery store, and the mall. Somewhere along one busy day, my Dad, who insisted on shoving the bottles into his jean pockets, lost the pain medication. The situation which ensued involved horrendous stress: driving to the hospital for another prescription, dealing with insurance, who would not cover another prescription so close to the last, waiting an hour for the busy doctor to write the prescription, then finding a pharmacy with enough pills in stock in conjunction with Dad suffering as I nearly pulled my own hair out trying to get the medication, and get it FAST!

That day, while in the pharmacy, I snatched pill boxes: the typical seven slot one, a three slot one, a ten slot one (for pills throughout the day), and a miniature one he could stick in his pocket. Just the other day at the pharmacy I found one that will attach to the car keys! The key chain pill box made me think of how we carried keys in college ~ we all had the long necklace key chains we wore around our necks and I thought of how I'm sure I could have talked Dad into securing a key chain pill box around one of those things we used in college! Pillboxes come with timers and alarms on them and nearly any size imaginable. Some of the key chain pillboxes I saw were even shaped like frogs and ladybugs, completely disguising the boxes!

After the pill box realization, I put a pain pill or two in a miniature pill box in the glove box, whoever took him to the hospital for treatment carried one in a purse on top of the ones he carried in that darn pocket! It also allowed him to put pain pills in pillboxes next to his bed, in the bathroom, in the kitchen and next to his chair. Be cautious of where the pillboxes are stashed if animals or children are around who could gain access to the medications.

I realize it seems an obvious, simple, almost unnecessary suggestion, but it is one that would have made my family's life easier through cancer that slipped our minds. Chemo brain among patients is a widely discussed phenomenon, however, as a caregiver, I called my "chemo brain" phenomenon "cancer brain." Cancer brain can cause relatively intelligent people to overlook simple solutions like pillboxes. A distressing experience arises when a cancer patient is even fifteen minutes from home (or two hours from home after leaving the medical center in traffic) and suffers because pain medication is needed and not available. The pain cycle, once in motion, becomes more difficult to crush. Remove the chance of suffering with pillboxes in your car, in your purse, in your pocket, on your key chain, etc. It is one simple step to improving life in the daily routine of cancer.

Chapter Seventeen ~ Good Vibrations

Make a hospital bed, hospital chair, family room chair, car ride or desk chair more comfortable. The week after my Dad's cancer diagnosis, I was out shopping for his upcoming birthday. I happened upon a cushioned back massager that plugged into an electrical outlet or a vehicle cigarette lighter. The cushioned seat strapped to the chair with elastic, heating and massaging the back and sitter. My Dad ended up with one in his office, one in his truck and one in his easy chair. Later, during outpatient chemotherapy, he appreciated the heat and massage on the drive home from chemotherapy. During the sixteen days in the hospital after surgery he had to get up and sit in a chair multiple times each day, and the heat and massage provided a pick-me-up and incentive for following through with the chair routine. Use any form of heating pad with caution during treatment though, as thinning skin increases the risk of being burned.

These massagers are available in department stores, bath and linen stores, superstores and even pharmacies. For prices as low as $20, the body can receive comfort and relief while it faces the fight-of-its-life. These stores also have tubs for heated water and massage apparatus' for sore feet, massage mats for the bath, massagers for the feet and neck and hand held massagers. For the ultimate in massage care, novelty and high-end product stores like "Brookstone" offer countless massage options. Comfort and massage are invaluable gifts for cancer patients. In addition to the natural desire for pain relief, feeling good and feeling free of pain helps the immune system build up defenses and lead the battle against those cancer cells.

Chapter Eighteen ~ Car Bags

The likelihood of nausea and vomiting often increases in the car. The motion coupled with a body undergoing cancer treatment make vomiting in the car a more likely possibility. To prevent messes, smells, discomfort, an automobile accident, spending time on the side of the road when you have to make it to the doctor's office and to ease the concern of vomiting in the car, carry bags in all vehicles. Shove them in the glove box, center consul, and cubby on the side of the door, in the pockets behind the seats or on the floor. Plastic grocery sacks will do the job, but double bag them. To avoid any possibility of holes, kitchen plastic garbage sacks work better and are very compactable. Make everybody's life easier and have bags on hand.

Driving down a busy highway with a cancer patient hanging out the window, fearing impending vomit, or a cancer patient stopping the car every 10 yards, feeling nausea spreading, or a patient vomiting all over the car because you couldn't get out of the fast lane in time, makes everyone's day worse. Vomit bags coupled with an extra set of anti-nausea acupressure wrist bands in the car can make the difference between a clean car and a vomit filled car. I stop and think of how sensitive my dad became to smells after different cancer treatments. The smell of my husband's cologne, the aroma of my gum, or take-out food in a bag in the back seat were all enough to make my dad gag and vomit. It drove him crazy, but there was no effective measure to take except having bags ready and waiting.

We have a video of my dad that I would insert as a video clip here if it were possible. My dad took a combat flying excursion as a birthday gift on several occasions. Inside the cockpit, cameras videoed my dad flying with an instructor. At one point during the turbulent fighter ride, the instructor offered over a barf bag. My pale, queasy looking dad shooed the bag away. As the instructor returned the bag to his side, with his body turned away, my dad gestures that 'oh, maybe I will take that bag.' The instructor misses the gesture, but on second glance, hands him the bag and tells him to put it over by him for safekeeping. Accepting the bag nonchalantly, he turns and pulls it open in a hurry, vomit apparently filling his mouth. Tough guy as he was though, he fights back the vomit and puts the bag away. That instructor probably knew the value of having bags on hand!

The likelihood of someone vomiting in his cockpit probably correlates to the likelihood of the cancer patient undergoing treatment feeling the urge to vomit at some point in the car. In the world of cancer, nausea and vomiting loom as ever-present possibilities, arising for nearly any reason at all. Packing bags will help everyone involved. My mom always said, "Better to never use them then need one and not have any!"

Chapter Nineteen ~ The In-Home Spa

Transform the bathroom into a mini get-away. For those days when energy stores have dropped below zero, every single thing about being around people has become irritating or house-atosis sets in, the bathroom can become a mini-spa. This tip goes for any member of those going through cancer: the patient, caregivers, family, etc. Candles, bubble bath, bath and shower gel, salts and oils and some music can help create an in-home oasis. Lavender or mint scented products aid in relaxation and soothing. Mint, whether peppermint or spearmint, and ginger act to curb nausea. Body stores often carry aromatherapy lines with sleep sections containing lavender or relax sections with spearmint and eucalyptus, in addition to other options. Products from health food stores offer more natural options for body products. The "Kiss My Face" and "Burts Bees" products contain very natural ingredients and have a variety of body care products to choose from.

One Christmas, when the department stores had all their cool electronic gifts on display, I found a portable, battery operated CD player that folded down and was barley larger than a walkman. It became the ideal CD player for the bathroom retreats after long days at the medical center, for soaking and sobbing, or just a good long hour of self-care! Now, radios that attach to the shower wall and iPod bathroom docks make music in the bathroom a piece of cake.

Simple comforts can make an enormous difference in mind and body health during cancer treatments for cancer patients and caregivers. Having items to aid in stress relief and comfort on hand can provide quick escapes without leaving the house at a time where often ones energy level keeps one at home. Bubble bath, candles, and relaxing music can all provide escapes. Long bubble baths, with lavender scented candles, and relaxing music were frequent escapes used after long hospital days at our home. Spearmint, peppermint or ginger candles and oils were frequently used when nausea and vomiting arose. Lavender relieves stress and promotes relaxation. Drops of oil in a bath or oils in oil diffusers help. Bath pillows, thermal bath spa mats, loofas and washcloths all contribute to the creation of comfort and relaxation.

Out of the bathroom, massaging foot spas, with or without water, can be used while sitting on the couch, relaxing in a lounger, or in a chair. Scented lotions, scrubs, and oils can all be used in conjunction with the bath or foot spa or on their own. A foot massage, shoulder massage, or scalp massage can make an enormous difference after a day with pain, exhaustion and stress. Keep in mind, though the use of candles can serve as a relaxing pleasure, candles burn up oxygen in the air and release carbon dioxide, so it is a good idea to use them in moderation, open the windows to allow fresh air in and consider adding green plants to the house to increase the supply of oxygen.

In my family, we can specifically recall the daily simple gestures we offered my dad that extended love and comfort. We rubbed his feet, massaged his back and squeezed his shoulders. We provided relief, distracted him from his pain and showed him we could sit beside him in his darkest times. There was no undoing the diagnosis, going back in time, or predicting tomorrow: there was simply the moment to be present with him, offer him the gift of love, and provide support during the cancer battle.

Chapter Twenty ~ Being Cuffed

Investing in a home blood pressure cuff allows for daily blood pressure monitoring or examination when feeling poorly. The side effects of chemotherapy, radiation and numerous drugs taken in the course of cancer treatment present dangers that carry the potential of becoming life threatening. Clinical trials also use drugs that carry serious side effects or unknown side effects depending on the level of the trial. When a patient feels poorly, a blood pressure device can allow you the power of numbers when calling the doctor. Moreover, blood pressure numbers are crucial indicators in determining whether an emergency room visit is necessary. Consistently high or low blood pressure readings in the doctors office may go unnoticed, thus taking the doctor a log to show daily numbers can be extremely useful and potentially lifesaving. Some new at-home blood pressure devices, available at most pharmacies, even have an automatic printer tape attached, further facilitating the process.

When my dad underwent new up-and-coming treatments, an array of serious and bizarre side effects occurred. Outbreaks, fevers, shivering and dizziness caused alarm. Monitoring his blood pressure helped us determine when he needed to go to the emergency room versus when we had things under control. His oncologist mentioned how incredibly useful it was when we began bringing him a daily log of his pulse and blood pressure through treatments. He exclaimed, "If all my patients did this, I could save more lives and provide even better care." Some of the reason patients are not bringing in logs of blood pressure is because they do not know how much it helps. I believe every patient wants to do whatever he or she can to have the best chances of beating cancer and improving his or her medical care, and this is one thing that will help. Patients going into cancer with a history of heart problems, or older patients may find this suggestion superfluous, something already a part of their daily regimen. For a patient like my dad, however, a young, perfectly healthy, tough guy, the thought of buying a blood pressure cuff did not arise until far into treatment.

Blood pressure monitoring takes a minute a day but could save a life. On the day of a cancer diagnosis, simple medical devices, like the blood pressure machine, should be required materials!

Chapter Twenty-One ~ When Temperatures Rise

Another necessity for surviving the cancer experience is a high-quality thermometer. We started out with a digital thermometer from the local pharmacy and quickly discovered it worked less effectively than the paper throwaway thermometers. The truth of the matter is, in cancer, a degree or two does matter. Thus, for the most effective readings, a highly effective thermometer is necessary.

The destruction done to the immune system by chemotherapy agents, radiation and cancer can interfere with the body's ability to regulate its internal temperature. In fact, cancer itself can cause a perpetual fever as the immune system battles cancer cells. Fevers in cancer patients can quickly cause dehydration and a host of other problems. Emergency treatment often becomes necessary. Each patient is different; each cancer is unique; and, each doctor follows slightly different protocols, so ask the doctor what temperature should drive you to seek treatment. While undergoing chemotherapy then clinical trials, my father had to seek treatment for any temperature. At other times, during treatment breaks, only higher temperatures required treatment. Fever works as an alarm system in the body; in general, a mild alarm; in cancer, a potentially serious alarm.

The time to buy a good thermometer is not when panic arises because a fever appears; the time is now, before any fever arises. Our favorite thermometer was the ear thermometer: it's fast, keeps the patient from having to put something in his or her mouth and is highly accurate. Supplies of disposable thermometers were also present as a back up at all times. Ear thermometers keep a patient from the danger of sticking a contaminated thermometer into the patient, and risking further infection. High quality, reasonably priced thermometers can often be found at wholesale retailers, superstores in addition to pharmacies and medical supply stores. Consider asking your doctor or nurse what type and brand of thermometer they recommend for home use.

Include the thermometer in a basket or cupboard where your necessary home medical supplies gather together, prepared to quickly help if needed.

Chapter Twenty-Two ~ Drug Lists

Lists of medication names and dosages belong in any patient and caregiver's wallets. Perhaps only two or three drugs sit in your medicine cabinet right now. Even so, those chemo-brain or cancer-brain moments may transpire out-of-the-blue and cause problems, especially if any emergency-type situation arises. As cancer treatment goes on, the list of medications often grows. Jot the medication names and dosages down on a 3x5 index card and stash it in your wallet. The list can easily be added to if and when the list lengthens.

Medications and dosages are vital for any doctor offering any treatment. If your medical center or hospital offers any massage, acupuncture or related type of service, they too require medication information. By ensuring medication names and dosages are recorded and in a patient's wallet, the information will most likely be available and found despite any situation that may arise. If an emergency arises and the paramedics are needed, the medication list will be available immediately whether the patient is conscious or unconscious. Considering all the situations that could arise: car accidents, fainting, seizures, choking, and falls, to name a few, not having a list of medications on your person could mean the difference between life and death.

Medication names and dosages must be available upon any doctor visit. Even at our monthly visits to the medical oncologist, the doctor who initially prescribed all medications, always began with listing medications and dosages, because the oncologist had to determine if any other physician prescribed additional medications. A list of two or three medications grew to ten or more depending on the week. In addition, a list of any over the counter medications, vitamins, supplements and herbs are necessities to take along as well. Soon, my dad's list of medications and supplements filled a 3x5 card. Our physicians greatly appreciated receiving a list of all the medications to copy down quickly rather than listening to us trying to recall all the medications, wasting both our time as well as that of our treatment team. Physicians do not know whom else you may be seeing and need all medications and dosages to offer you the best treatment.

Carrying a list of your medications and dosages will expedite treatment at the doctor's office or hospital, ensure your safety and guarantee the best possible care.

Chapter Twenty-Three ~ Take Back the Power

Before signing up for a clinical trial, investigate clinical trials available for your specific type of cancer and specific current health status in your area, nationwide and beyond at www.cancer.gov/clinicaltrials and www.clinicaltrials.gov. There you can investigate the possibilities available before committing to a specific trial. Often, the matter becomes rather simplistic because prior treatment, surgery and diagnosis, coupled with current health status can quickly limit the number of available trials. Moreover, searching oneself allows more control and choice than if otherwise just placed in a pool of clinical trials by a physician or cancer center.

When my dad reached a point where conventional treatments had been exhausted, he was placed in the cancer center's pool of available clinical trials. Then, he began a Phase I Clinical Trial. A number of clinical trial options existed at that point throughout the country in which he met the criteria for. Some were in Phase II others Phase III. The higher the phase number, the longer the drug has been tested, and the more promising the outcome often seems. In our case, cancer was far advanced, moving proved highly implausible, as all his physicians for palliative care and pain management were at this cancer center, and moving would have seriously threatened his well being. I emailed the principal investigators of a number of trials in several different states and countries. I was pleasantly surprised when I received highly informative, empathetic emails in return to my inquisitions. The emails of the principal investigators are available at both www.cancer.gov/clinicaltrials and www.clinicaltrials.com.

In retrospect, I somewhat regret not choosing a different trial that was further along in development, available an hour away, which sounded more promising. At the time, we needed to act quickly and time was of the essence. Basically, if deciding to pursue the clinical trials avenue, make sure you feel comfortable with the trial chosen, as the process can prove grueling. Funding is limited, disorganization often creates frustration and much more patience is required than in other treatments.

My father took part in a Phase I stage of a new, promising drug by an impressive developer. The trials required him being in the hospital for twelve-hour stretches of time for observation. Scheduling and poor organization of the clinical trial department led to his initial treatment beginning seven hours later than originally scheduled. Resultantly, we were driving home from the hospital at one o'clock in the morning. This would have been a one-time frustration had we known that once beginning, a precise schedule had to be maintained, thus treatment lasted until 1am for several weeks. For a pain-inflicted, suffering, weak cancer patient, who joined the study after drawn from a clinical trial pool, the lack of control and frustration mounted.

Clinical trials exist to further the success of treating cancer, with the aim of eventually curing cancer. Stop and consider that the drugs of today, curing and prolonging the lives of those with cancer, were all in clinical trials at some point in the past. Every participant matters and plays a part in making a difference in the future of cancer treatment. Feeling as though you still have control and say over your treatment is a crucial aspect of your treatment and life. Check out the clinical trials websites and take comfort in the number of choices constantly available.

Chapter Twenty-Four ~ More Record Keeping

Doctor appointments often consist of a rapid flooding of information, results, options, treatments and courses of action. Recalling all the information accurately after leaving the doctor's office can prove challenging. I recall walking out the door, answering the phone to repeat the information just shared in the doctor's office and feeling blank: like the doctors appointment was a month ago, or perhaps I daydreamed it happened, or it could be my mind was left in the consultation room. Therefore, I began relaxing, taking a tape recorder in, and having the appointments taped. Any physician carrying out his or her position appropriately should readily consent to the taping of appointments. Oncologists stretched thin attempting to help a sea of cancer patients and extreme stress accompanying the doctor's office, create an environment where information shoots off in rapid succession, making recording hand-written notes challenging.

When my mom learned of my dad's cancer diagnosis, she was in a busy waiting room expecting uneventful results of an upper endoscopy done because of frequent hiccups. She could barley understand the doctor through his thick accent, let alone anything else. The weeks after the diagnosis were filled with appointments: perspectives on surgery versus no surgery, chemotherapy choices, radiation philosophies and hours of doctor's appointments. One day the problem was the hiccups, the next day he was given 15 months to live. Recalling and later regurgitating facts, statistics, drug names, complicated procedures and specifics of his devastating news proved an impossible feat. So much of what happened that first week is gone; stress and trauma permanently erased what doesn't exist in medical files.

I recall attending doctor appointments with him much later, when recurrence surfaced. The prestigious and sought after physicians were sure to spend as much time as we needed. I believed I understood and would recall what the physicians said, however, I think the hallway out of the doctors office had some invisible devise that sucked out memory and details. Without the tape recorder, half the doctor appointment was gone by the time we stepped foot out the door. Time and again I found accurate recollection was only realistically attainable by using a tape recorder.

Accurate written records of each doctor appointment, indicating change in treatment, prognosis, diagnosis and treatment plan, are guaranteed only when a tape recorder dictates the news back to you later. These recordings prove extremely useful at the beginning of treatment, as the shock and overwhelming news of cancer pollutes the memory. Having a precise transcript to reference when comparing differences and similarities in opinions from professionals and recalling crucial aspects of appointments may make the difference in the outcome of treatment. Often terminology used prevents absolute understanding in a doctor appointment, unknown drug names and procedures may pass without a patient catching an accurate note, and certain specifics, which seem clear at the time, dissipate later. We live in a day and age where contacting the doctor is becoming more of a challenge. Everyone involved would rather you have the tape to reference than have to call the doctor for a refresher on what he or she already said. Additionally, keeping appointment recordings empowers and enables the patient to have more control over his or her cancer treatment.

In the beginning, shock and emotion may fog recollection; however, as time wears on, the cancer process in itself erodes memory, making the tape recorder just as important later in the cancer journey. The historical nature of the recordings provides testimony to what one survives through. Tape recorders now come so compact, comparable to the size of several stacked credit cards, making their portability and simplicity easily manageable. Any doctor refusing a tape recorder in his or her office would send me running!

Relieve yourself of unneeded pressure and burden and take a tape recorder with you to doctor appointments. It will prove an effortless way to simplify the cancer experience.

Chapter Twenty-Five ~ Pain Busters

Pain of muscles, joints, bones, headaches, backaches and comprehensive body aches seem part in parcel of cancer treatment at one time or another. Amazing topical pain allies available for experimentation are *White Flower Analgesic Balm* and *Tiger Balm*, available everywhere from health food stores to drug stores.

White Flower Analgesic Balm contains wintergreen, menthol, camphor, eucalyptus, peppermint and lavender. It is commonly used for headaches, sinus problems, aches and pains caused by rheumatism or trauma, stiffness, poor circulation, sore muscles, blood stasis, swelling, arthritis, neuralgia and lumbar pain. *White Flower,* my personal choice, consists of a liquid that one rubs onto the afflicted area. As a sufferer of migraines for years, I find relief by rubbing *White Flower* over my scalp, neck and shoulders. *White Flower* has dramatically altered the course of headaches and migraines in my life by offering an instantaneous help in great pain while my migraine medication takes action. The only English words on the packaging the product comes in are *"White Flower Analgesic Balm,"* but don't let this keep you from experimenting with the product.

Tiger Balm offers versatility, coming in many different forms, making it great for many different types of pain and diverse preferences. *Tiger Balm* has a line of balms, patches and liniment with various sizes, making transporting the product simple. Herbalist Aw Chu Kim asked his sons Aw Boon Haw and Aw Boon Par to perfect the product after his death in the 1870's in Burma. Thus, today Haw Par Healthcare manufactures and distributes the product. Contents consist of menthol, camphor, beeswax, petroleum jelly, oil of clove, oil of cajuput, oil of cinnamon and ammonium hydroxide (ammonium hydroxide is in the red product line only.)

Both *White Flower* and *Tiger Balm* are comprised of natural oils and herbs; however, it is always important to carefully read the ingredients, warnings and directions before using these products. Also, when receiving chemotherapy and radiation, the skin can become thin and highly sensitive, so these products should be tested on a small area of skin before applied generously to the body. For instance, for me, the strong strength of *Tiger Balm* leaves dry, red marks on my skin that feel like sunburns. *White Flower*, on the other hand, only slightly dries my skin, but the relief outweighs the disadvantages for me.

The premise behind *Tiger Balm* and *White Flower* mirror those of more commonly known analgesic rubs found in grocery stores and pharmacies, however they are comprised of more natural ingredients and are better suited for widespread body use. *White Flower*, for me, proves a pocket-sized powerhouse against pain. I use it for muscle aches (and can attest that the product should not be used on newly shaven skin), headaches and muscle tension. Little bottles of *White Flower* remain in the bathroom, kitchen, desk, purse and car at all times. The instant relief offered by the *White Flower* feels like soaking my entire head in a large bucket of ice, or a spa soak to achy legs. The strong mint aroma also tends to curve nausea.

These products can quickly, effectively and naturally ease suffering and pain. Try *White Flower Analgesic Balm* and *Tiger Balm* and see if they improve your quality of living and decrease your quantity of pain.

Chapter Twenty-Six ~ Secure Your Scans

Imagine sitting anxiously, with news of metastasis, with a patient in pain, hearing that scans packed away in a hospital basement two thousand miles away are needed immediately. Palliative radiation to ease incessant pain made the scans an urgent necessity. What transpired next was flying to California (otherwise the hospital would have needed six weeks for the records to be excavated, sent, and received in the right place), renting a car, finding a hotel room, talking to a nurse about getting the scans, searching out a doctor who would go over the nurse's head, after she said it would take a week to get the scans, actually getting the scans, then flying two thousand miles back with the scans (after facing insistence that the scans be placed in luggage and checked-in), and waiting for another doctor's appointment to evaluate the scans. All the meanwhile a cancer patient sought more and more pain medication to ease the suffering of a growing lymph node pushing on a nerve.

The preceding story could have been completely avoided had we gathered all scans, reports, x-rays, and records before heading off for treatment at a different hospital. Unfortunately, in the tornado of terror when the news of recurrence arrived, nobody thought to go gather scans at the hospital. We thought all the records we had were good enough. In the midst of an oncology team deciding cancer treatment should begin two thousand miles away from home in two days, my parents left for treatment, as my 18 year-old sister and I packed up our home, and moved everything in the course of about two weeks. While packing from dawn until dusk, nobody considered the scans from radiation would ever become a necessity, until that day, seven months later, while my dad suffered.

If I had walked into a fortuneteller while we still lived in California, and the fortuneteller would have told me that my family would be moving two thousand miles within the year, I would have laughed hysterically as I retold the story to friends and family later. My point being: the unexpected happens; and happens more frequently than not in the world of cancer. Plan for the worst; expect the best. My father's treatment began at a cancer center ranked within the top 10 in the nation. We were beyond confident in the treatment options and plan. Recurrence, however, set into motion a new dilemma. His treatment team said there was nothing more they could do. Meanwhile, another top ranked cancer center said they had several options left and should begin treatment as soon as possible. It turned our lives upside down, and that is the essence of what the experience was like, beginning to end: as soon as we thought it was under control, it mutated, changed, and we had to find an entirely new strategy for handling it.

Gathering reports and blood work immediately following every procedure gives a patient the upper hand in the process of having all his or her information if a second opinion becomes necessary at any point. Scans, unlike reports, remain the property of the treating institution. After a CT scan or PET scan, the patient should obtain a copy of the report, detailing the findings; however, the actual scans typically remain at the hospital. This is changing, however, as more institutions gain the capacity to place the scans on a DVD for the patient. Upon having an X-ray, MRI, CT scan or PET scan, ask the technician, physician or nurse if obtaining a copy of the scan on DVD or CD is possible. This will dramatically hasten care and treatment. For instance, in my experience with sinus trouble and surgeries, I paid five dollars each time for a DVD of the scan. Although, I learned usually the hard copies of the scan itself remain best; having the DVD's with me bumped up the time frame I received treatment and surgery in. Rather than running the test again, as often occurs, the physician could quickly reference my DVD and return with an opinion.

If DVD or CD copies have yet to become an option at your hospital, the scans can be checked out. Whether you have DVD or CD copies or not, hard copies of radiographs absolutely should go with a patient if he or she visits any other hospital. Moreover, in checking the scans out, they usually say the scans must be returned within a specific period, however, I have never had any hospital call to get their scans back. The waiting game, attempting to track the scans down in the midst of pain and suffering, is beyond nerve wracking.

The risk of getting the scans and ending-up over-prepared far outweighs having to painstakingly wait for the scans to arrive if they become instantly necessary. A time or two, I received comments or strange looks, nurses saying, "Nobody's ever asked for a DVD copy of their scan before." This is a contributing factor to why patients are dying accidentally and unnecessarily: because self-management of ones own health care is not sufficiently and enthusiastically encouraged. People do not operate under the "do not question, do not take charge" motto in general day-to-day living, ones body and healthcare should be no different.

Scans prove especially indispensable in the case of radiation, because a maximum dose of radiation exists. Once one body area has received a maximum dose of radiation, the area cannot receive more radiation. The scans are the only way of precisely pinpointing what exact area received the dosage of radiation specified in a report.

Excessive radiation can result in death; therefore, having the scans to reference could mean the difference between life and death.

Prepare for the unknown, expect the unexpected, and gather every piece of the treatment record before heading off for a second opinion or new treatment.

Chapter Twenty-Seven ~ An Oral Offense

The human mouth is a moist, nutrient filled, warm environment: the ideal habitat for bacteria. Helpful and harmful bacteria enter the mouth easily and readily everyday. The threat of bacteria becomes a more serious issue during cancer and cancer treatment. Using Biotene mouthwash throughout the day has numerous benefits for the cancer patient. First and foremost, it is an antibacterial mouthwash, free of alcohol, with four natural antibacterial enzymes that kill bacteria found in oral infections. Keeping bacteria low in the mouth improves the chances of remaining healthy during cancer treatment.

In addition to warding off bacterial infections, rinsing frequently with an antibacterial mouthwash helps dispel oral fungal infections. The white fuzzy fungus that commonly plagues the tongue and cheek after chemotherapy may not appear at all if rinses occur frequently throughout the day.

Frequent mouth rinsing also helps aid in dry mouth problems that arise as side effects from chemotherapy and radiation. Dry mouth, more than an irritation, can give rise to the biological imbalance that allows a bacterial or fungal infection to occur in the mouth or more extensively in the body. A dry mouth is characterized by a sticky or dry sensation in the mouth, problems with chewing, swallowing, tasting and even speaking, bad breath, burning sensation in the mouth, cracked lips, a dry tongue, mouth sores, sleep interference, gum inflammation, and infection in the mouth. The three pairs of salivary glands create a protective system in the mouth, and when chemotherapy and radiation disrupt the salivary system, a crucial antibacterial defense system loses power. *Biotene* contains three enzymes and one protein found naturally in human saliva, helping to restore and protect the natural oral balance in the mouth, keeping the antibacterial system in the mouth functioning properly. Natural enzymes Glucose Oxidase and Lactoperoxidase work together to generate a flow of hypothiocyanite ions, strong antibacterial agents that must always be present in saliva. Additionally, Lysozyme helps split the cell wall of pathogenic bacteria and Lactoferrin inhibits pathogenic bacteria by denying them iron. Together, these natural ingredients work together to promote and create a healthy, moist mouth, free of bacterial and fungal infections. In addition to restoring a natural, healthy oral environment, *Biotene* is free of alcohol and strong flavoring that creates stings and burns found in other mouthwashes.

Consider keeping a variety of sizes available. Large bottles work well for the bathroom, as small bottles allow for easy transport. Keep a steady supply of small bottles for transport during long hospital days, travel, work or time spent away from home. Consider packing bottles away with the rest of your cancer care kits in a purse, bag, glove box, toolbox or pocket. You can even reuse the little bottles, refilling them using the large bottle.

My dad kept bottles of *Biotene* handy and took them with him more than any other single item when going to the hospital, whether for an inpatient stay or a long day of treatment. He never developed oral fungal infections when he consistently rinsed his mouth. Interestingly, he never got a single cold, virus, flu, etc. through cancer treatment, even when his white cell count dropped too low to do treatment. Actually, when his white cell count dropped lower than it had ever been, we went to *Graceland*, Nashville and *Disney World*, and he still managed to remain totally healthy. He did religiously ascribe to two simple, useful antibacterial measures throughout treatment: he used his antibacterial mouthwash frequently and kept his hands clean.

Add antibacterial mouthwash to your daily routine. Develop a habit of rinsing your mouth with a quick squirt every time you use the restroom. Keeping the mouth clean, moist and healthy is a first line of defense in keeping the body healthy during cancer treatment.

Chapter Twenty-Eight ~ The Cancer Preparedness Kit

You need an updated, stocked, first aid kit when headed into the cancer battle because the only thing one can certainly expect during cancer is the unexpected. Hydrogen peroxide, *Betadine* solution, antibacterial cream and gel, rubbing alcohol, latex gloves, cotton swabs, cotton balls and bandages must remain in stock at all times. The slightest cuts should receive adequate disinfection during cancer because chances of infection increase when immune system response decreases.

My dad arrived home from surgery, after sixteen days in the hospital, with eleven wounds where holes, cuts and incisions were healing. The hospital wanted them frequently swabbed with *Betadine* solution and re-bandaged. We realized none of these things we needed were on hand. The same thing happened when he had a jejunostomy tube re-inserted much later in treatment. Finally, the second time around we wised up, gathered adequate supplies at the pharmacy and kept them in a first aid basket for easy access where they would remain together.

Cleaning any wound with hydrogen peroxide or *Betadine* solution while using a cotton swab or cotton ball decreases risk of adding any bacteria to the area by applying the solution with a sterile material as opposed to something like toilet paper that hangs next to the toilet, gathering particles of fecal material every time the toilet is flushed. Variety packs of bandages allow adequate preparation for any cut or incision. During one round of treatment using a biological therapy and chemotherapy, my dad developed sores over his face, hands and head. They induced the greatest pain on his hands where they infested all his cuticles. Bandages of many different sizes were necessary to treat all the different wounds.

Latex gloves should cover any hands tending a cancer patient's wounds. Grabbing a sterile cotton ball with glove-free hands contaminates the cotton ball, in turn, potentially contaminating the wound under care. Latex gloves can make the difference between an infected wound and a properly healed wound. Latex gloves were always part of the first aid basket at our house. Twice my dad had a jeujunostomy tube: once for all nutrients and hydration, then later for caloric contribution to the diet. He had a tube inserted in his side, where a clearly open wound remained. He needed water and food through this tube. Any time the tube was handled at all, even by his hands, even though there was no direct contact with skin or the wound, latex gloves were an absolute necessity.

When battling cancer, the immune system is needed for building new healthy cells, restoring the body to health and fighting a life-saving battle. One must fight to avoid adding increased demands to the system, or from developing infections by defensively treating wounds in a more aggressive fashion than the average person not going through cancer treatment treats wounds. Gather the first aid supplies now, before an open oozing cut has to wait for someone to make a trip to the pharmacy.

Chapter Twenty-Nine ~ Prevent Infection

Antibacterial soap and gel keep hands clean and further decrease risk of illness and infection. Some soaps lack antibacterial properties and are rather useless for killing bacteria. If antibacterial soaps abound in a cancer patient's home, the patient, the patient's family and visitors to the patients home kill germs removing threats to the patient's health. The Center for Disease Control and Prevention (CDCP) says the single most effective way to prevent infection is washing hands. The CDCP stresses the importance of removing jewelry, using warm water, rubbing all surfaces of the hand (front, back, wrist) for at least fifteen seconds, rinsing, and then drying off the hands with a paper towel, shutting off the faucet with the paper towel and opening the bathroom door on the way out with the paper towel.

More germs are transmitted via hand contact than any other mode of transfer. I cough on my hand (politely covering my cough) then reach down and open a door, hit a light switch, flush a toilet or turn on a faucet, leaving my germs to lay in wait for when you come along and open the door, turn on the light, flush the toilet or turn on the faucet. Then you reach for gum, unwrap it, drop it into your hand, and pop it into your mouth. For this reason, hospitals and medical professionals stress washing hands frequently. Posters in many cancer centers suggest it's actually unkind to shake hands. Hand shaking gives one more avenue of disease transfer!

One of the kindest things loved ones can do around cancer patients is wash hands, wash hands, wash hands. Using antibacterial hand gel when washing hands is impossible (such as on a plane, in the car, in a store) keeps the hands adequately sanitized when away from the bathroom. The CDCP also recommends an alcohol-based rub. They advise massaging it on all hand surfaces until the skin dries. Antibacterial hand gel is another item stashed in every corner of our environment: by the remote controls, in the kitchen, in the office, in the bag that goes to the hospital, in the center console of the car, etc. It is an absolute necessity!

Consider frequently disinfecting the locations in your home swarming with germs. Places that receive high hand traffic should undergo recurrent disinfection. Disinfecting spray or wipes should swipe door handles, light switches, faucets in the kitchen and bathrooms, the handle that flushes the toilet, television remotes, handles to the refrigerator, microwave, oven, dishwasher, pantry door, frequently opened drawers and steering wheels at least daily. I made an afternoon and late night swipe through the house, using a different wipe on every surface frequently touched by hands. Beyond the previous list, I included the piano keyboard, computer keyboard and mouse, stair handrails and window latches. A recent commercial illustrated the germ danger, with hands touching things through the kitchen and then showing the surface of the object as if under a microscope, with bacteria looming over surfaces. When dealing with illness prevention during cancer, we should look through eyes that can imagine what surfaces look like under microscopes, disinfecting commonly touched surfaces thus decreasing the threat of spreading infection through your home.

Out in the natural environment, hand sanitization becomes an even higher priority. Because of thinned skin resulting from cancer treatments, we insisted upon my dad carrying latex gloves to wear when putting gas in the car. The number of people, sick and healthy, who touch those pumps everyday, which go un-sanitized, is staggering. The grocery store carts loom with thousands of germs. The pin pads where you swipe your credit cards, or the electronic pens, or the pen the checker hands you to sign with, all have been touched hundreds of times each day. Community pens, like those available at the bank, door handles into stores, check-out counters, and any other frequently touched surface, hold bacteria, awaiting the transfer to the next pair of host hands. These are the cases that make the antibacterial gel beneficial and useful. The dilemma during cancer becomes the extremely weakened state of the immune system, and therefore the prevention of unnecessary illness. Beyond the common cold, there are all kinds of people, from all over the world, meandering through the grocery stores, malls and restaurants with all kinds of illnesses.

When white blood cell counts plummet, doctors recommend facemasks and gloves. This prevents acquisition of airborne illness, and picking up illness from hand contact. Under chemotherapy and radiation, whether white blood cell counts have plummeted or not, prevent against germ invasions. Washing hands with antibacterial soap and using antibacterial gel for the cancer patient and family are part of a first line of defense for keeping oneself healthy during cancer, hopefully even preventing the glove stage.

Chapter Thirty ~ Masquerade

Facemasks abound in cancer centers. Historically, physicians and nurses sported masks in the operating room, to promote a sterile environment, until it dawned on someone that cancer patients can effectively keep themselves free from many airborne pathogens by placing a surgical facemask on when entering highly populated areas. Still, often masks are only utilized when patients have low white blood cell counts; however, facemasks should not be limited to low blood-cell counts or to the hospital. Children are big germ carriers, as are many cancer patients with compromised immune systems.

The masks can mean the difference between catching a cold and remaining healthy if forced, for one reason or another, to remain in an environment with sick people. Perhaps you want to catch a movie, but coughing people surround, or perhaps while waiting in an emergency room, you realize many others are there with infections. Having a mask available can ease the mind and create a barrier between you and lurking infections. I was able to find packs of fifty for about ten dollars at the nearby medical supply store.

One unfortunate reality affecting cancer hospitals is shingles. We experienced a bout of this through cancer as well. One difficult aspect of shingles, the virus more commonly known as the chicken-pox virus, varicella-zoster virus, is its highly contagious nature before an outbreak is detected. Shingles is a threat to those who have not yet had chicken pox and pregnant women. One imagines, while sitting in a hospital waiting room, perhaps the emergency room, or perhaps waiting for blood to be taken, a person with shingles would be recognizable, however, as the actual blisters begin in warm places on the body, they can be easily hidden by clothing. Face masks, along with latex gloves and antibacterial gel help to protect oneself from threats like shingles to the immune system.

In some places, such as airports and airplanes, a patient is practically asking to catch something without taking precautions such as wearing a facemask. In places like our airports, where funding is spread so thin already, machines, chairs, etc., are not being disinfected frequently enough to keep one healthy! The hospital, bank, post office and pharmacy are other locations filled with sick people, children and germs. High bacteria counts have been found in bathrooms and on money, but also in movie theaters, kitchens and grocery stores! The cancer patient practically has to train the naked eye to imagine bacteria present so as to remain healthy.

It also becomes necessary for the patient's caregivers and anyone living with the patient to perform a risk analysis for him or herself. Considering that the added stress of cancer affects caregiver's immune systems, their risk of catching colds also increases. For instance, in the face of cancer, my mother found herself catching frequent sinus infections when flying. The germs in places like airports should cause those close to the patient to evaluate his or her own needs for prevention. If sick and in the same home with a cancer patient, a facemask acts as another level of protection. The guilt created by passing a cold onto a cancer patient makes one cringe!

Flu season is a threat to cancer patients as much as sick people who certainly will be in any environment you go into. Unfortunately, they leave behind their bacteria, viruses and sickness. Even once they have gone, the threat silently lingers. Pack a facemask in a purse, bag or pocket as an option in highly populated areas. Better to get a look or two than an illness, perhaps a trip to the hospital, or anything to drain your immune system during the fight of your life. During cancer care, germs cannot be out-of-sight, out-of-mind.

Chapter Thirty-One ~ Acupressure to the Rescue

Acupressure wristbands work miraculously against the side effects of cancer treatment. A circular plastic piece presses on a pressure point on the wrist, decreasing or obliterating nausea and vomiting. My dad, a built, muscular, tough-guy, began wearing them during his first treatment after a rough first day. They almost instantly ended the nausea and vomiting. He never left for chemotherapy again without them on! And he never experienced vomiting as a side-effect again. He was not one for the alternative treatments to nausea: the mint teas, or peppermints, or ginger. The acupressure wristbands, though, were rather permanent fixtures.

The *Sea-Band* brand has stood strong against clinical testing and proved to decrease, prevent and reverse nausea caused by travel, pregnancy, anesthesia, chemotherapy and other conditions that typically induce nausea. The band utilizes acupressure principles, offering a drug free alternative for situations where nausea and vomiting occur. Moreover, the bands are free of side effects, a main difference between the wristbands and their drug counterparts. The pressure exerted on the P6 acupuncture point on the wrist relieves both long-term and short-term nausea. If nausea has already begun, the bands can become effective within five minutes. The bands can safely be worn around-the-clock and in any setting. Consisting of mixed fibers, and free of latex, the bands are comfortable, washer safe, long-lasting, safe to wear in the shower, pool or any body of water and conducive to any wrist size. Investigate yourself the brands that have specifically undergone clinical testing. The testing caused me to reach for the brand name variety in the pharmacy.

The bands typically come in a light blue color and are available in most pharmacies, usually alongside the seasickness medications. Considering their inexpensive, non-drug, non-invasive nature, they are certainly worth a try for anyone. Chemotherapy can be unpredictable: the first, second, and third rounds can go fine, then the fourth round suddenly produces severe side-effects: the course depends completely on the individual, the specific agents and the dosages. No two people respond exactly the same. With that said, the acupressure wristbands have worked for us more consistently than an array of anti-nausea medications. And they work quickly! We ended up with the bracelets stashed, in their small plastic boxes they come in, everywhere: cars, purses, bags, drawers, by the TV remotes, in the kitchen junk-drawer, in an overnight bag, in a main tool box: you get the idea. In consideration of the price of the drugs that worked to combat the nausea, the price of the bands was miniscule and well worth it. I say, don't leave home to chemo without them!

Chapter Thirty-Two ~ Cancer Specific Meditation

Dr. Bernie Siegel, the founder of *Exceptional Cancer Patients (ECAP)*, surgeon, author of Peace, Love and Healing and Love, Medicine and Miracles and inspiration to millions, sells meditation tapes specifically for cancer patients. The number of available tapes and CD titles continues to expand, each as spectacular as the last. Bernie's meditation tapes, available in bookstores or online, provide instant, tailored meditation for cancer patients. Rather than stopping to learn meditation in the midst of a diagnosis, doctor visits and treatments, I opted to pop Bernie in the tape player. I became addicted and now have trouble making it through my day without him or sleeping without him, although he recommends the meditation be used at intervals through the day in an alert state, rather than a sleep state. I carry a portable cassette player and pop the tapes in for a ten to fifteen minute meditation when necessary.

In the fear, exhaustion, stress and pain of cancer, I find Bernie Siegel's meditations critical daily treatment. Comprehensive cancer treatment centers often offer meditation as amounting research accumulates on the benefits derived from meditation. Buddhist monks were studied in a monastery in northern India. While practicing meditation, Tibetan monks, wearing very little, sat still and unaffected in a room set at forty degrees Fahrenheit. I can barely ski decked out in ski clothes, in forty degree weather! Some monks were covered in sheets soaked in forty-nine degree Fahrenheit water. For most, these temperatures would induce shivering, and possibly, if body temperatures continued to drop, death. The monks had steam rising from the sheets and dried three sheets each. At Harvard Medical School scientists are demonstrating that meditation can relieve suffering in cases of illness and stress. Meditation practices are being studied and shown to decrease stress and illness among all types of people and lifestyles, including cancer.

Dr. Siegel's meditations include titles such as: "Meditations for Finding the Key to Good Health", "Getting Ready" (geared toward preparing for surgery, chemotherapy and radiation), "Meditations for Morning and Evening", "Meditations for Overcoming Life's Stressors and Strains", "Meditations for Difficult Times", "Meditations for Peace of Mind", "Healing Meditations", "Meditations for Enhancing Your Immune System" and "Meditations for Everyday Living." My favorites are "Meditations for Difficult Times" and "Healing Meditations," but I have them all and they all come highly recommended. I strongly recommend trying out one of the tapes, perhaps even "Meditations for Difficult Times", for the cancer patient and his or her family. Feel how the body responds. These meditations could be one of the greatest gifts you offer a cancer patient, caregiver or family member. Bernie's heart for cancer patients reaches out from these tapes to embrace the listener and ease the suffering and stress illness has on the body and mind.

Chapter Thirty-Three ~ Active Participation

Dissent is actively discouraged in many hospitals. Hospitals, in their endless devotion to treat as many patients as possible, have to reward and reinforce passive compliance. In an institution where the professionals are swamped with patients, with so many sick people that they do not necessarily need your business, patients often receive the message to keep quiet. Keep at the forefront of your mind that you are receiving treatments from fallible human beings, not perfect machines. Speak up when you have questions. Actively insist on receiving information until you feel comfortable. Force the physician and/or nurse to answer all questions. *You have the right to say no!*

At one of the best cancer hospitals in the nation, I watched my father passively fulfill the role of the "good" patient, requiring one of us there with him to prevent mistakes. Once he had a catheter in his arm, delivering a radioactive substance for an imaging procedure. I left for the rest room and came back to find his arm swelling. Panicked, I asked what has happening and he assured me it was fine. I ran from the room for help: obviously it was not fine. He told me, "I just figured they knew what they were doing." The needle popped out of the vein and was filling the skin with the substance. His arm hurt for a week afterwards!

Another time my dad was in the hospital, having just had a jejunostomy-tube, a feeding tube that is inserted into the small intestine, surgically placed. That morning the doctor from his clinical trial came in and, with a team of physicians, decided against delivering the trial agent until he recovered from surgery. Later that day an intern arrived to give him the trial drug. Half asleep in the chair beside his bed, I bound to my feet barking, "No, there's been a mistake." This lady pushed closer to my father, handing him the cup, and I pushed closer, taking the cup. The man was loaded full of pain medications and an intern rushed in and continued boldly overruling me as though I was hallucinating when I quoted the clinical trial team. To make a long story short, this nearly turned into a "chick fight" (as my dad called it) right there in the hospital room! But it could have been a serious and costly mistake! Many study drugs carry the threat of death and laying there anorexic, weak and in pain, he could have become one of those statistics. The clinical trial department was so overworked that we had to become an around-the-clock team of patient advocates for one patient! When I stop and consider what could have happened if I was out stretching my legs when the intern came in, I cringe!

Since that time I have heard one story too many about mistakes leading to suffering, illness and even death. I certainly believe health care professionals are doing their best to follow protocol and orders; it is simply a busy, stressful environment for everyone. One would most likely argue if you walked into a pharmacy, asked someone stalking the shelves for a pain reliever and were handed Vitamin C. Medical degrees, nursing degrees and internships do not place people above the capability of making mistakes or above questioning. I have tremendous respect, admiration and appreciation for all my father's brilliant physicians. But I believe the best realize they really are humans in white jackets! Human beings make mistakes. My experience only makes me confident in questioning even the doctors who do not want me questioning them; especially the doctors who don't want me questioning them! Question! Speak up! It could mean the difference between life and death.

Chapter Thirty-Four ~ Got Pain?

A great tool in pain management is the Transcutaneous Electrical Nerve Stimulation (TENS) unit. Unfortunately, this non-drug, non-invasive tool is under utilized and not known widely enough. Even a world-renowned oncologist and his assistant asked what it was! It consists of four electrodes placed strategically on the body, connected to a patient-manipulated, battery-operated, pack about the size of a cellular phone.

The device works by sending electrical impulses through the electrodes placed on or near the painful site. The pulsations interfere with the pain message arriving and registering in the brain. The TENS unit also helps increase the release of endorphins, the body's own natural painkillers. The patient experiences a mild, comfortable tingling sensation. Carrying very few risks, the TENS unit can act as a powerful tool in pain management for cancer patients. The TENS unit should not be used by patients with pacemakers, unless otherwise instructed by a physician. Also, the electrodes should not be placed over the carotid sinus, meaning anywhere on the front of the neck. One of the most important aspects of pain management is breaking the pain cycle and the TENS unit is renowned for its ability to break the pain cycle.

The TENS unit requires a prescription. Just as medications, they are typically covered by insurance and yet very reasonably priced to begin with. I used a TENS unit after a back injury and found great relief from its usage. My father received a TENS unit for back pain cause by an enlarged lymph node pressing on a nerve. When his first line pain medication began failing, the TENS unit provided tremendous relief, allowing him sleep, when pain medications and sleeping medications were failing him. My only regret is that we didn't ask for one much, much sooner! It wasn't until his pain specialist recommended it that we reprimanded ourselves for forgetting about it.

Got pain? Get a TENS unit!

Chapter Thirty-Five ~ The Alternative Medicine Bibles

If you have the slightest interest in alternative additions to your treatments or alternative treatments in themselves, the book Prescriptions for Nutritional Healing: A Practical A-to-Z Reference to Drug-Free Remedies Using Vitamins, Minerals, Herbs and Food Supplements by Phyllis Balch is a must have. In my father's case, six weeks separated the doctor's visit to the first chemotherapy treatment, by no choice of his own. It is difficult to sit back and "do nothing" and simply wait. We promptly implemented every suggestion from Prescriptions for Nutritional Healing for cancer. He joked because all the vitamins caused him to burp puffs of "smoke" (vitamin powder). Does that sound alarming? No more alarming than vomiting, hair loss and anorexia, common side effects of chemotherapy and radiation. Certainly it is no scientific study, but from the time of his first endoscopy to the endoscopy before chemotherapy began, the tumor went from being the size of an apple to the size of a walnut!

An example of information you might come across in Prescriptions for Nutritional Healing involves one of my favorites currently being widely researched in cancer: curcumin. Curcumin, a component derived from the Indian spice turmeric, has demonstrated anti-inflammatory effects and research has demonstrated it prevents cancers and can inhibit tumor initiation, promotion, invasion, angiogenesis and metastasis. This Ayurvedic agent has been demonstrated to alter over 700 different genes. Curcumin blocks the production of tumor cells, induces apoptosis (a cancer patients favorite word, meaning the process by which a cancer cell commits suicide), prevents the conversion of a healthy cell into a malignant cell, inhibits invasion and metastasis and curbs inflammation. It is important to note that questions remain as to whether curcumin interferes with chemotherapy or radiation; therefore, you should consult your physician before deciding to take curcumin. Some health conditions also make taking curcumin a risk. Consider checking the websites of prominent cancer centers that can lead you to sections that explain recommendations and warnings with vitamins, herbs and supplements. Put curcumin in the search box and you can find possible interactions and health conditions that may make taking curcumin a risk. My favorite resource sites for supplements come from www.mdanderson.org and www.mskcc.org.com.

Finding a rather safe spice shown to have similar affects as biological therapies and chemotherapies is promising and exciting in the cancer world. Curcumin and other promising agents fill the pages of Balch's book. Phyllis Balch now also has a number of other books to consider in addition to this title as collaborations with other authors. Consider adding these books to your library. Remember to always consult your physician before beginning any new vitamin, herb, supplement or other protocol.

Chapter Thirty-Six ~ Pharmacy Phone List

Consider calling your pharmacy or the pharmacies near you before leaving the hospital with prescriptions to fill. For a great deal of time we had no issues whatsoever because the largest big chain pharmacy in the area was a block from our house. A little later in treatment, however, we ran into a massive dilemma that taught a tedious and stressful lesson. We arrived home from the hospital at seven or eight o'clock in the evening with a load of prescription slips. We hit the pharmacy, and as I previously advised, I asked the pharmacist to ensure they had the drugs before we left. She was not amused; neither were the people behind us in line. They only had one or two of the drugs! This should have been alarming, but at the time I was unaware that it was the largest pharmacy in a twenty-five-mile radius. I spent the next four to five hours pharmacy hopping.

The story is long and useless to repeat. The concluding moral of the story is that there are some medications nearly impossible to get except for at the hospital! I had pharmacists telling me 'this medication doesn't come in that form' and 'this state doesn't sell that medication.' One pharmacist suggested I make a twelve-hour drive to a neighboring state for the medication! The truth is, some cancer medications are intense and dangerous and often even large pharmacies do not want to assume the liability of having them in stock. This seems particularly true of liquid pain medication, or rather liquid forms of any medication that a child would not routinely receive. Liquid medications can become necessary in cancers where swallowing or eating is an issue, or where medication can only be delivered via tube. Moreover, for the first time, I discovered that pharmacists can be highly misinformed about the existence of some drugs. Three different pharmacists told me that the drugs prescribed did not come in the prescribed form under any circumstances. Moreover, they were highly convincing, searching giant encyclopedia like books and databases. I sat arguing, asking, "Why would world renowned doctors prescribe medications that don't exist?" The pharmacists maintained their position. They were telling me he would just have to take the oral form. I explained, "He cannot swallow, it's impossible!" And they acted like I was just trying to be difficult for the fun of it. This was simply one more lesson in the specifics of cancer treatment that nobody tells you about!

So, finishing my hellish pharmacy tale, we ended up going through the night without the medications and spending half of the next day at the hospital obtaining the prescriptions. It turned out the doctors were not wrong, the pharmacists were wrong. Never again did we go home without a) filling our prescriptions at the hospital, or, b) calling our neighborhood pharmacy to make sure they had the drug, in the prescribed form, on hand! Find three large local pharmacies and program their numbers into your cell phone! Don't wait for the one night where this story happens: prevent it now.

Chapter Thirty-Seven ~ The Portacath Debate

Portacath's provide intravenous access for patients requiring frequent or continuous administration of intravenous substances. They allow for output, such as blood draws, and input, such as chemotherapy. After diagnosis, an outpatient surgery was promptly scheduled to place a portacath in my father's upper right chest. This little rubber ball laid under the skin and allowed a major vein to be easily accessed for drug delivery, blood draws, anything usually requiring consistent needles in the arm. At the time we were told that since chemotherapy often wrecks havoc on the veins, a portacath keeps the veins in the arms from being destroyed during chemotherapy. We were told it would be surgically removed after chemotherapy.

After chemo, radiation and surgery there were arguments between doctors over the portacath. One said, "Take it out"; it required monthly maintenance and can become infected.

Another said, "Leave it in"; you never know when you will need more. In the end, for either no reason or reasons I have forgotten, it stayed.

When we switched hospitals, the new hospital adamantly opposed using portacath's and the portacath actually complicated treatments. A special nurse, someone trained in accessing the catheter, had to be paged any time it was used, lengthening wait times. Moreover, I sat and listened to horror stories of infected catheters. At one point, signs suggested a hidden infection lurked and the first line of defense was going to include removing the portacath. At the time, my dad suffered with shingles, metastasis, and anorexia. Serious concern heightened over whether he would survive the surgery required to remove the catheter. The portacath became a lurking ominous fear. Nobody ran through this possible case scenario the day they implanted it.

Risks other than infection exist with portacaths. A blood clot in the catheter may permanently block the device, known as thrombosis. Monthly maintenance when the catheter is not in use, involving a flush with saline and heparin, occurs to prevent the blood clots. Mechanical failure of the device, although extremely rare, also exists as a possibility. Finally, a collapsed lung and artery damage remain as possible side effects. To be fair though, the portacath is highly convenient and prevents skin and muscle tissue damage caused by chemotherapy.

Ask for the positive and negative, the views on both sides of the catheter debate before going through with it. In the end, if the catheter would have needed to be removed when it was thought to be infected, I am certain I would be an adamant opponent to the portacath today. In reality, it turned out fine and removed the necessity for needle pokes and finding veins. Investigate the debate: the decision deserves serious thought.

Chapter Thirty-Eight ~ Bowel Obstruction Prevention

An unfortunate side effect of many cancer medications and treatments is bowel problems. Bowel-obstruction patients consistently fill the emergency rooms of cancer hospitals. Pain medications are a top culprit but not the only drugs to blame. Pain medications slow down the movement of the stool in the intestine and remove large amounts of water from the colon. Patients often avoid this uncomfortable topic of conversation with their physicians. Additionally, doctors sometimes fail to stress the serious nature of bowel obstruction. At the height of pain medication regimens in our house, three different types of stimulant laxative and stool softeners were utilized many times a day. Even then, enemas were necessary. Brand names in the pharmacy, available sometimes at the grocery store as well, are a much better, less painful alternative to hospitalization for bowel obstruction.

How often is necessary? A bowel movement is necessary everyday. Otherwise, the build up of toxins in your system leads to an array of serious problems. As unappealing as enemas are, I imagine a visit to the emergency room for bowel obstruction (often requiring surgical intervention) to far exceed enemas on the scale of unpleasant experiences.

Doctors recommend many over-the-counter treatments in addition to prescription choices. Over-the-counter laxatives and stool softeners were frequently recommended by a number of doctors we saw. There was also consistent agreement that using brand name enemas sold at pharmacies on an as needed basis to prevent constipation is rather safe. Note that when blood counts are low enemas cannot be used. Ask your doctor what laxatives, stool softeners and enemas they recommend.

Be sure, in the meantime, to drink at least two quarts of fluid a day and keep a healthy amount of fiber in the diet. For fiber in the food source, incorporate whole-wheat breads, wheat cereals, wheat bran, rye, rice, barley, most other grains, cabbage, beets, carrots, Brussels sprouts, turnips, cauliflower and apple skin, for insoluble fiber; oat bran, oatmeal, beans, peas, rice, bran, barley, citrus fruits, strawberries and apple pulp for soluble fiber. For supplemental fiber, many brands available in the grocery store and pharmacy offer the flexibility of multiple sources: capsules, stir in powder or liquid, or even tasty wafers.

Whole psyllium husks, available in health food stores have no sugar, gluten, sweeteners, colors or additives. Whole psyllium husks not only support regularity and ease elimination, but also remove toxins, improve digestions, lower elevated cholesterol levels, balance blood sugar levels, reduce diarrhea issues and promote colon health. Most people bathe, brush their teeth and brush their hair everyday. Psyllium husks are like an internal brushing and cleansing. Keep in mind it is absolutely necessary to drink plenty of water when taking any fiber supplement. Moreover, psyllium, present in most any fiber supplements, should not be used with bowel narrowing or obstruction. Also, any fiber supplement should be consumed several hours away from medications as they can delay the absorption of medications.

Check with your doctor before adding any stool softener, laxatives or fiber supplements to your diet. Also, check with your doctor as to whether you can safely use enemas. I spent an hour too many of my life in doctors offices talking about the crucial nature of daily elimination.

The horror stories in the emergency room made me ask, "Why aren't patients consistently being told of the dangers created by letting elimination difficulties go untreated?" Bowel obstruction is risky and unpleasant business. Keep it regular!

Chapter Thirty-Nine ~ Comfort Treatment

Soft things make a dramatic difference during cancer. Blankets, bathrobes, slippers, sweat suits, socks: all things extremely soft, add significant comfort during this stressful battle. *Brookstone* makes a collection of blankets, bathrobes, bears, slippers, pillows, etc. in their *n.a.p.* collection that are extremely comfortable. They feel like cuddling with a golden retriever puppy! Linen and body stores sell ultra-soft robes. I recently found a robe that zips up the front and stops just below the knee in addition to a variety of other soft robes I collect for comfort. Slippers and socks abound that are so soft it's like walking on clouds. Cashmere socks, available in department stores, feel like a foot massage! Even superstore chains carry soft blankets, robes and socks for just a few dollars. These creature comforts can bring sighs of relief during twelve-hour days at the hospital, inpatient chemotherapy, or days where side effects knock a patient to his or her knees. Personally, I love Jersey cotton sheets: a mixture between cotton and flannel, with down throws. Home stores are full of things for all rooms of the house that will bring comfort and great temporary relief. These home stores abound in great gift ideas for cancer patients and cancer caregivers.

During chemotherapy and radiation, skin cells face destruction, increasing sensitivity to touch. A soft blanket to a cancer patient can feel like a bubble bath or mud soak. The simpler things in life, like soft tactile comfort, can make a massive difference in physical, emotional and psychological well being during cancer.

Chapter Forty ~ Tricks to Stop Nausea

Stash mint flavored things in quick access places: in the house, car or purse. Mints, gum, peppermints and things of that nature often help stop the sensation nausea blankets one with and can prevent vomiting as well. Mint teas are often recommended as well, however I find drinking mint teas when feeling nauseous can often place something in the stomach to vomit up and then the teas can become aversive or even develop an association with vomiting. Others find great relief from the frequent use of mint teas. I find mint tea the most helpful before the sensation of nausea sets in, as a preventative measure. The mints in the mouth or mint gums, as they don't pour liquid into a queasy system, work well too! I use spearmint gum with great success. In the worst-case scenario, the mints can ward off vomiting until one gets out of a public place or out of the car.

Ginger is also held as a powerful anti-nausea remedy. *Altoids* makes a ginger flavored mint, containing real ginger. Ginger teas can lead to the same results and associations as described above. Shredded ginger root in the mouth can help, but if swallowed and regurgitated, it can cause a burning sensation in the esophagus. Ginger tablets might be something you consider adding to your regimen before treatment or throughout the day. Adding fresh ginger into foods or teas may work to prevent nausea and vomiting.

After a great deal of experimentation, I dive for the mints, but I would guess by the research on ginger, that it probably works well in combating nausea and vomiting for many people. For reasons of promptness and practicality, have rolls of mints, tin boxes of mints, or packs of gum stashed in the kitchen, bedroom, bathroom, by the TV, in the car, in a pocket, bag or purse.

Chapter Forty-One ~ Bead Packs

Heating pads impart an additional threat to patients, as cancer patients face increased risk of receiving burns. A perfect alternative is the microwavable bead pack. Options include those with aromatherapy herbs and flax seed beads or unscented specialty beans. Stores specializing in back care products often sell unique types such as those with elastic bands with Velcro, so the pack can be strapped on, leaving one free to walk around without trying to hold the pack in place; or those with soft, fluffy covers. The up-sides to the microwave/freezer packs compared with the traditional electric heating pad are the obvious versatility, the different shapes and sizes for different body parts and the herbs inside, like lavender and mint, adding to relaxation. Herb choices include: chamomile or spearmint as relaxants, peppermint, rosemary, lemon grass or white willow as pain relievers, saw palmetto berry for rejuvenation, valerian root works as a calming antispasmodic, yellow dock root improves circulation, lavender relieves headaches, migraines and pain, cinnamon as an antispasmodic and yarrow to promote healing.

The packs originally came in a rectangular shape perfect for lying on or draping across the abdomen. Now, at our house, we have one the size of a lap blanket, multiple typical rectangles, one designed to lay comfortably over the shoulders, small rectangles designed for the face and head, and even socks, slippers and gloves! Others I have seen include those inside stuffed animal puppies, kitties or teddy bears. Online I found a wrist wrap, elbow wrap (capable of helping any joint) and lower back wrap. Search herbal heating pads or bead heating pads in a search engine. These packs add great comfort and relief through cancer. It was our consistent experience through cancer that if my dad was in pain or uncomfortable and we asked if he wanted a pack, he usually said no. But if we popped them in the microwave and then laid one over his shoulders or legs, he would always tell us how greatly it helped! We even had a designated pack that went to the hospital on treatment days that gave him great comfort there too!

Keep in mind the small eye packs, socks and mittens usually only go in for 30 seconds. Also, the burning smell that happens when the packs spend more than 2 minutes in the microwave can burn holes in the pack on top of smelling atrocious! A pack being reheated should only spend 30-45 seconds in the microwave to avoid this burning! If your microwave does not have a turntable, or the pack's size prevents it from turning, flip the herb pack over half way through the heating process to avoid burning the pack. Misting the herb packs before microwaving them will offer moist heat to the user in addition to bringing out the herb scent, while prolonging the life of the enclosed herbs. If you do not have a microwave, or do not use a microwave, the packs reportedly can go in the oven for 15 minutes at 350 degrees, however they need to be wrapped in foil and should be placed on a pan. For freezer use, Ziploc bags should encase the bean pack.

This tool can also travel to the hospital as well, for use while in treatment or while waiting in doctor's offices. Every doctor's office and treatment wing I even spent time in had a microwave. All places where chemotherapy was administered had microwaves for patient and caregiver use, making repeated warming of the bead packs a piece of cake. Be weary of knock-offs or cheap substitutes: some contain barley and rice, which do not absorb or offer heat. Please note to share the warmth with caregivers! This is another great gift idea for cancer patients and their caregivers. We never seem to have enough of them at our house!

Chapter Forty-Two ~ A Written Legacy

Bookstores, card stores, large pharmacies and sometimes even grocery stores and large pharmacies carry these great memory books. The books I prefer, by J. Countryman, are entitled <u>A Father's Legacy,</u> <u>A Mother's Legacy,</u> and <u>A Grandparent's Legacy</u>. They become an easy companion for chemotherapy days or down days. These question and answer books require the reader to fill in questions like: "What is your favorite childhood memory," or "Tell me about when you met mom." My dad filled in a good portion of a book for us. Another option I've seen, for people who resist filling in the pages (or just plain refuse to do it) is asking the questions and video taping the answers, or having the listener fill in the answers. These memory books are a great way to create unforgettable moments with your loved ones. Rather than sending a message that they won't live, it is sending a message that his or her life story is important and the legacy book turns an individual story into history, capable of being passed down.

My dad was a big storyteller, and without him here to repeat the stories, I've forgotten some details. I am so happy to know there is a place I can find the details! I recall one night when his health was deteriorating rapidly and we all felt grieved and frightened. Because of the book, we asked for a story from his childhood. He started on about journeys with his friends in Indiana onto the army base at night. "We would create adventures and sleep out there."

"When you were 8?" we exclaimed.

"Ya," he answered.

"You just slept on the ground?"

"Sure" he answered his amused city girls.

"What did you eat?" we asked.

"Fish," he said. "We'd catch fish and eat them."

"You made a fire and cooked them?!?!"

"Sure," he smiled.

"How did you cook them? On sticks or something?"

He stopped and thought about it.

"Well, usually we took cans of beans and weenies," the story changed.

"And you just ate them cold?"

"How did you open them?"

"You took a can opener?"

"And a pan to cook them in?" we took turns jokingly badgering him.

Finally, a smile spread across his face, and a quiet laugh changed the story. "Why do you guys ask me to tell you a story, just to ask a hundred questions about it?"

"Well, we're trying to accurately set the scene in our minds," I answered.

As more fact crept into the story, he admitted,

"Well, we'd stay out there if we had some blankets", and, "We would take matches and start a fire, and bring cans of beans and weenies, open them with a pocket knife, warm them over the fire, then eat them." This night of simple stories was a moving night of connection close to the time of my dad's death that I remember with great warmth.

The memories shared in these books far exceed any other thing that can be passed down. Cancer brings the issue of ones mortality to the forefront and so now is the time to start recording your own individual, unique, never-to-be-repeated, life story to pass down. Pass it down now or 80 years from now. It can't be passed down if it's never written down!

Chapter Forty-Three ~ Massage On The Go

Portable, battery operated, hand-sized massagers are available in pharmacies, home stores, department stores and even some grocery stores. They are portable, inexpensive and useful. We toted one along in our "chemo bag" every week to chemo days and even doctor visits. During rough chemotherapy days, running the massager on my dad's back, down his legs or arms, made a big difference. It requires little effort for the operator, can be used by the patient on him or herself, and offers great relief.

Massage is utilized more and more in cancer institutions throughout the country. Massage, capable of decreasing anxiety and depression, and increasing endorphins, the body's natural painkillers, works to distract the mind and relieve physical pain. At both cancer centers we experienced, mini-massages were offered, free of charge to patients receiving chemotherapy with permission from the treating physician. Massage offers relaxation, stress reduction and distraction from pain. The fun massage trinket offers a variety of different options to the patients now. Many brands offer simple, lightweight, three pronged, hand-held massagers that run off batteries. There is also a flat hand held massager covered with a soft material, non-battery operated plastic massage instruments and other new trinkets appearing everyday.

Tote a mini-massager to the hospital, chemotherapy or even in the car and see it make a positive difference in pain, stress and discomfort.

Chapter Forty-Four ~ Shower Power

Shower chairs remove all effort from showering. My dad was adamantly opposed to a shower chair until the day I brought one home and said, "Just try it and if you don't like it, we'll get rid of it."

That night he exclaimed, "I should have gotten one of those the day I started treatment! I might never leave the shower again." For patients drained of energy by treatment, the shower chair, available at any medical supply store, allows a person to remain in the shower without fears of slipping, falling, fainting, or just expending the little energy left on a shower. Fatigue and lack of strength accompany most cancer treatments. The shower chair not only acts to prevent injury, but also gives the patient access to luxury: a nice long shower while kicking back in a chair. Hospice introduces shower chairs upon coming into a home, and I see no reason to wait for hospice to get a shower chair. They simply make showering simpler and safer for any person low on energy. The clean, refreshing, rejuvenating feeling of bathing can provide a boost in itself. The shower chair increases this beneficial experience.

I remember being in the medical supply store and debating the purchase with the storeowner. "What's your return policy?" I inquired.

He asked, "Why would you return it?"

I explained, "My dad's a big tough guy, who is neither old nor terribly sickly, but he is low on energy and strength and I worry about him. Last night he was afraid my husband was going to have to pull him out of the bath!

But there's a good chance he is going to refuse to have anything to do with this chair."

"Why do you say that?" he continued.

My husband laughed, "Because he told her not to go buy one."

This large, athletic, muscular man in his thirties said, "I have a shower chair in my house. I just kick back in there and relax with my coffee." It was more information than I needed, but his wife confirmed he loved his shower chair!

I decided to sneak the chair into the shower and hope when he went in, the chair wouldn't come flying out into the hall…. It never did, he fell in love with it and regretted not making his life easier much sooner!

About a month later, I returned to the hospital supply store. "I don't see the chair," the storeowner said.

"Nope, I'm back for something else," I said, continuing my shopping.

"He loved it didn't he?" he shot back.

"Ya, you were right."

"I always am on the shower chair," he answered. "Nobody has even asked about returning one before you."

Some shower chairs come with wheels, so a patient can be transferred from a chair or wheelchair and wheeled right into the shower. They come available as simple as plastic chairs not damaged by water (for this type a cheap outdoor chair could do the job), compact plastic chairs for small shower space, to as complex as chairs with leg, arm and head support. Consider the shower chair as a gift for any cancer patient.

Chapter Forty-Five ~ Pressure Sore Prevention

Pressure sores, more commonly known as bedsores, should remain constantly in the mind of anyone facing cancer, in addition to caregivers. Believe it or not, they can become a big problem for the patient even knocked-out or tired from chemo for one week a month. Continuous pressure reduces blood supply, leading to death of cells, skin deterioration and thus the creation of open wounds near bony areas on the body. The back of the head, back of the ears, shoulders, tailbone, spine, elbows, buttocks, inside of the knees, ankles and heels are common sites for bed sores, proving painful, constantly irritated, areas. They are painful, can become infected, are difficult to treat, and slow to heal because of damage to the immune system by cancer treatments. They disturb sleep, upset comfort and are overall unpleasant.

The trick to avoiding bedsores is simple: one must decrease pressure to the same areas of the body. Hospice recommended we have him move every fifteen minutes. This suggestion for an uncomfortable cancer patient in pain proved totally impractical. Also, an air mattress is often recommended. My dad felt less disturbed by us adding egg crates to his bed and his chair: the two places he spent the most down time. The egg crates help distribute the pressure of body weight more to prevent bedsores. The egg crates are comfortable: add them before the bedsores ever appear! Slipping down in a hospital bed or chair also helps contribute to the sores, and the egg crates help prevent the sliding.

Additionally, adequate protein consumption and sufficient hydration play a part in preventing pressure sores. Another consideration is skin hydration. Use lotions to properly moisturize the skin. The hospital environment brutalizes the skin, as the low humidity, which helps prevent the spread of infection, removes moisture from the skin, drying it and making it more prone to breaks and cracks. Keep the skin healthy using gentle, natural lotions.

Keep the possibility of pressure sores in the forefront of the mind throughout treatment and prevent them. We were never warned of the possibility of pressure sores. For my father, the sores were a constant source of irritation, frustration and discomfort. I feel very sad just remembering the time when bedsores became one more problem to address when he suffered greatly. The contributing factors of weight loss, skin cell destruction (from chemo and radiation), decreased mobility, increased sitting and inadequate nutrition led to the development of pressure sores before anyone could find warning of these issues.

If this section came too late and bedsores are already present, be sure to point them out to the doctor. They need to be treated with antibiotics, kept clean and adequately tended to. Often patients omit information from their physician because the bedsores often arrise on the buttocks or tailbone; however, this is a mistake as infections can grow and threaten the patients overall well being. If left untreated, a bedsore could land you in the hosptial. If at all possible, prevent pressure sores now, before one more added stressor and discomfort becomes a part of your cancer treatment.

Chapter Forty-Six ~ Cancer Adventures

Adventure: an exciting or very unusual experience; participation in exciting undertakings or enterprises; a bold undertaking. These definitions only begin to define the wonderful events that transpired in our lives during cancer: our treasures from cancer. Every family and every cancer patient desires the end of cancer to include recovery and healing, above all else. Regardless of the cancer type, stage, metastasis, age, or any other factor, each person realistically faces his or her mortality: the reality that now or later, life ends. The certainty that is left, that which can exist whether cancer regresses or not, is adventure.

My family's cancer experience is unique. Physicians, psychologists, grief counselors, and others have consistently remarked, "Your story is amazing. Hardly anybody spends that much time together." Many times we hear, "You really did it right," and, "So much of the time the pain and fear keep such great memories from being created." Our goal was never to "do it right," or anything else. Our family of perfectionists couldn't do cancer perfect, there's no such thing. Instead, we put one foot in front of the other, and persevered every step along the way (while great pain, worry and sadness provided continuous hurdles).

We set out to make memories, have fun, and create adventure. At no point was it a conscious decision, that, "Well, whatever happens, we'll have the adventures," but that is the reality we're left with in the aftermath of cancer. Scrapbooks overflow with the memories. They range from simple beach days together, that turned into tender memories, conscious attempts to make father's day or birthdays days to remember, to grand vacations.

The reason we found the usually undetected cancer, I insisted, was so my dad would be cured. He was very, very young. In retrospect, I believe the reason cancer was discovered was to give us all the memories. We all lived a very busy, nose-to-the-grindstone existence before cancer. My parents ran a successful commercial construction company together. My sister was senior of the month in high school, where she took the most advanced classes, played on the tennis team, took piano lessons and ballet lessons, to name a few. I was busy in grad school and working with autistic children.

Cancer stopped nearly everything in our lives dead in its tracks. All meaning changed, our focus shifted one hundred and eighty degrees from long-term goals to short-term goals. Life at six o'clock at our house one day involved Dad working in the garage, mom working in her office upstairs, my sister doing homework in her room while I studied in my room. The day after cancer arrived, we were all having dinner around the table, talking, like most people would be if we weren't so caught up in tomorrow and the future.

If the focus shifts from paralyzing fear over whether cancer will offer 50 hours or 50 years, to taking adventures together for whatever time life offers, the result will always be fantastic and perfect. In the midst of adventure, we are all really alive, while we remember all there is to live for.

My simple adventure memories remind me of walks around the bayou. One day, after chemotherapy, I insisted we go out to stretch our legs. My dad skipped singing, "May The Bird of Paradise Fly up Your Nose" just to entertain me!

"Dad," I said with embarrassment, "Control yourself."

"You said I was being a downer," he joked back.

For a few moments, he walked calmly beside me, pushing my dog's stroller (yes it's ridiculous, but she quits walking whenever she's done, sometimes leaving one stranded). As a bicyclist approached, calling out "On your left," I barked "Dad! Bike!" And he leisurely moved to the side. I shook my head disapprovingly. "You don't get how chemo brain sets in. That guy probably figured you were deaf because you reacted so slow." He didn't see how much chemotherapy made him so slow to think and react sometimes.

We proceeded along on the asphalt pathway. "Relax girl," he joked with me. We talked about how nice it felt to be out of the hospital, car and house and out walking around the bayou.

"There was really no place at home that we could get into a place that felt like we were off hiking in nature so fast," he remarked.

"I know, we'd always walk along those busy….."

As I spoke a bicyclist approached. "WATCH OUT, MOVE IT," my dad called, shoving me off the path onto the grass, nearly running me over as he shoved the dog's stroller over so as not to obstruct the bicyclist's path.

"DAD!!!!" I called out, laughing hysterically.

He was hysterically cracking up, doubled over with laughter.

"The bicyclist almost fell off his bike!" I exclaimed.

"Well, I didn't want chemo brain to make me stand in the road like a deaf dumb dope," he joked.

"You always have to go over the top," I said.

"That bicyclist jumped worse than you did!" he explained, "I think you've got some form of chemo brain!"

I can remember every second of that walk, though it probably only lasted twenty minutes. Neither of us had much energy. Both of us just needed some fresh air. But it was pure adventure (mostly created thanks to my dad!).

Then, I can hear Patsy Cline's "I Go Out Walking After Midnight (Searching For You)", but the voices singing are his and mine. Sitting outside the Ryman Auditorium in Nashville, the original home of the Grand Ole Opry, Mom practically shoved the two of us out of the car and insisted we go record a CD together in a recording booth in the Ryman. He recorded "Heartbreak Hotel" with my sister and, in his Elvis voice said, "Thank-you, thank-you very much," at the end of the song. To have our voices recorded together, singing, after all the years of loving music together, is such a moving memory to have now.

Or, I can contemplate our journey, fleeing two hurricanes, up to Graceland, Hurricane Mills and Nashville, then down through Tennessee and Georgia, into Florida. In Orlando, we played like kids together in the Universal Studio theme parks, and Disneyworld. One night, in the Magic Kingdom, we all rode "It's A Small World" together. A tourist sitting in front of us took about two hundred photographs during the dark ride, nearly blinding us. My dad jumped off the boat when the ride came to an end, and pretended to be blind, running into things and holding his hands out in front of him to help him feel his way around. My mom, sister and I laughed hysterically watching him. The tourist didn't seem to catch on. As he got on "Dumbo", he posed for a picture sitting next to my mom, making a face of terror, like he was crying, like a little boy. It's one of my favorite pictures I will ever own of my parents! We watched the firework show "Wishes" together, and were so moved, we all shed a tear or two. Of course, we realized we were all wishing for a cure.

Adventures are the real cure in cancer. Everybody wins, the outcome is always priceless, and the memories live on forever.

Chapter Forty-Seven ~ Medication Administration

A simple fact that may make a big difference in your cancer treatment at some point is that most medications come in many forms: pill, dissolvable pill, injection and liquid form. My dad faced terrible pain swallowing pills everyday for about two months when cancer reached advanced stages. Rather than a doctor changing the method of delivery of the meds, he suffered. I simply did not know that methadone and dilaudid came in liquid form. You can't pick them up at the corner pharmacy, but they come in liquid forms. For the last two months of my Dad's life, all his medications were in liquid form, and the two that were not, were crushed and mixed with water. Do not attempt to crush any medication without both the prescribing physician and the pharmacist's approval. Not all drugs can be crushed.

We reached a point where my dad could swallow nothing and panicked. But panic was unnecessary. Medications can be delivered via injection and via tubes as well. A feeding tube can be inserted specifically and exclusively for medication delivery, if you wish. Patches can be applied to different parts of the body for many different types of medications. Many drugs come in a dissolvable form as well. Doctors can keep physical pain away. If your doctor will not help, find a new doctor.

Chapter Forty-Eight ~ Treatment Entertainment

DVDs, CDs and videos speed-up that treacherous hospital time that seems to pass so slowly. While serving as distractions, they can change moods and ease pain. Norman Cousins sited the power Marx Brothers films made on illness in his life. "I made the joyous discovery that ten minutes of genuine belly laughter had an anesthetic effect and would give me at least two hours of pain-free sleep," he shared. "When the pain-killing effect of the laughter wore off, we would switch on the motion picture projector again and not infrequently, it would lead to another pain-free interval."

My dad's first chemo treatment involved inpatient, twenty-four-hours-a-day, intravenous drip chemotherapy in the hospital for seven straight days. His very first week of inpatient treatment was scheduled one week before his birthday. Accordingly, as an early birthday present, we purchased an inexpensive DVD and video combination player. We were able to hook the player up to the television in his hospital room. That hospital now brings back clear memories for me, one of bringing him the DVD Jackass on a day where rain poured and he was in the hospital. Doctors and nurses ran in throughout that hour, alarmed at his profuse laughter. Other favorites of my dad's were movies with Tom Hanks, Blazing Saddles, The Three Stooges, and Mash episodes.

After surgery he was in a shared room and the portable CD player allowed him to put headphones on and listen to Bernie Siegel's meditations and music. He closed his eyes, pushed play and escaped the hospital. In shared rooms, where one television must be shared between two patients, consider a portable DVD player (available in some places for relatively reasonable prices).

Later, at one cancer center, the rooms that outpatient chemotherapy is given in each have their own DVD and video combination machine. We would take 2 DVD's and my dad would always remark, "That went fast today." It was amazing that eight or twelve hours felt fast for him ~ it was the DVD player! With a portable DVD player, iPod, portable CD player or laptop, even waiting in the waiting room becomes much less of an issue. Entertainment is surely a necessity in the long hours that cancer treatment brings.

Chapter Forty-Nine ~ A Healthier Mouth

At superstores and discount warehouse stores you can purchase packets of 6-10 toothbrushes. Buy a pack or two and have new toothbrushes on hand. We wouldn't reuse tissues and expect to heal, consistently re-infecting ourselves, or use the same cup or fork for a week, and yet we hold the toothbrush to different rules. If you want to get healthier faster and keep from re-infecting yourself, follow stringent measures to keep your toothbrush disinfected and clean. A dry toothbrush does not equate to a germ free toothbrush.

Keeping a toothbrush clean can be accomplished by a variety of measures. Begin by washing your hands well before handling your toothbrush for any reason. Then, evaluate the options for storing the toothbrush in a germ free environment. Storing ones toothbrush in a closed container, in a solution of three percent hydrogen peroxide will kill off most pathogens. The hydrogen peroxide solution will need to be replaced after each use, and the container holding the toothbrush and solution should be washed frequently in the dishwasher as well. Soaking the toothbrush in mouthwash will kill off most germs; however, the safest measure would involve keeping the toothbrush in hydrogen peroxide everyday and dipping it in mouthwash in a disposable cup for thirty seconds before use.

Whether or not you choose to store the toothbrush in hydrogen peroxide, the toothbrush should be kept in a container, where contact with toothbrushes belonging to others does not occur. If the toothbrush is not stored in solution, then the container needs to be dry and the toothbrush needs to be totally dry before entering the container. Failing to store a toothbrush in a dry container may lead to mold growth and will certainly lead to bacterial growth. Just as a container with hydrogen peroxide, a dry container also needs frequent visitation to the dishwasher. Actually, the toothbrush and its container should frequently run through a dishwashing cycle, placed on the top rack to prevent melting. If the patient develops mouth sores or any cold or illness throw away toothbrushes frequently.

I had a series of sinus surgeries in college. After each one I would develop massive sinus infections that no antibiotic touched. Amongst awful nasal irrigation, downing the strongest antibiotics, spraying all sorts of things in my nose, I still could not get better. It took about ten ear, nose and throat doctors before someone inquired, "Do you change your toothbrush often?" They recommended I change it daily and I finally got better! It perplexes me why this isn't recommended to cancer patients, as they face increased risk of infection and work so hard to ward off infection.

Moreover, consider the placement of your toothbrush. During cancer treatment, with a compromised immune system, one must keep their toothbrush as germ free as possible. A toothbrush should not be left out on a sink if a toilet is in the area. Flushing toilets in the bathroom can lead to microscopic fecal material being on your toothbrush. Clever little containers for the toothbrush are not a simple solution as they rarely ever are dry, and thus provide the optimal breeding grounds for high numbers of bacteria and mold. For some reason, the change of the tooth brushing routine seems like a lot of work to some. Ignoring adequate care of the toothbrush is an odd part of many individuals routine if you consider most our habits. The health department checks restaurants and grocery stores to ensure proper cleanliness exists. We wash dishes, silverware, our bodies, and our clothes on a daily basis. The toothbrush though, gets stuck in a fangled toothbrush holder, sticking up to gather bacteria, or facing down to touch other toothbrushes and stays in a damp, wet cup. We stick the same thing in our mouth for months at a time, expecting running water over it to make it clean. This is another clear illustration of where we could use bacteria-vision goggles. Try to imagine how crawling your toothbrush can be, and the threat it presents without adequate daily upkeep and frequent changing.

What's the best solution? I'm unsure. I still change my toothbrush everyday! Studying microbiology will bring more worries than you ever hoped to have!

Chapter Fifty ~ The Light at the End of the Tunnel

A time may come when someone suggests nothing more can be done. This could be in reference to surgery, chemotherapy, radiation, pain treatment or all conventional western medical treatment. Start with obtaining a second opinion. If the second opinion suggests the same as the first, consider seeking a third. There is always something more that can be tired, there is always hope, there are always possibilities. There are people out there being told to go home and die. Things like "Essiac", curcumin, green tea, the macrobiotic diet, colonics, meditation, and literally hundreds of other things are reportedly saving lives every day.

Our original medical oncologist, one of the most prominent and finest on the west coast, said there was no additional treatment my father could receive, thus making a PET scan useless. Luckily, the surgeon and the oncologist were in disagreement. We followed the surgeon's advice instead, and had a PET scan. We left the state to visit the surgeon, who had since moved to another hospital. The PET scan lit up, indicating cancer. It was a devastating blow. We thought we were on vacation, stopping by to see our beloved surgeon, and then suddenly we were moving halfway across the country. The medical oncologist there insisted a number of treatment options remained available and started him on a new protocol the next day! The first medical oncologist said, "All we can do now is just keep him comfortable."

The second oncologist offered, "There are many options available to us. Let's get to work and see what we can do. And it's just my intuition, but I have a good feeling about you." Then my dad lived an entire year longer.

When I reported the oncologists' quote to the surgical oncologist, his jaw dropped and he exclaimed, "You're kidding! He's usually really cut and dry, more so than Dr. H" (Dr. H being the original oncologist). Giving up is never necessary! There are too many unknown factors. So many new and yet unstudied agents out there are making a difference. Until conventional science can obliterate cancer, I turn a rather deaf ear to their criticism of "alternative medicines," especially in situations where conventional medicine can do no more. No human being can accurately predict or even estimate the amount of time or degree of health any individual's life will have.

While I have witnessed the powers of chemotherapy in obliterating cancer, I simultaneously have watched the brutal side effects. Our conventional western approach to killing off all cells to destroy cancer cells is a bit like the old practice of "bleeding" people to heal them. In light of this, integrative medicine and alternative medicine deserve a podium in the world of cancer treatment. It makes little sense why we often turn immediately to western medicine, blowing off alternative medicine in westernized societies. Practices that comprise parts of what we refer to as "alternative medicine" include Chinese and Ayurvedic treatments that have been in use for over a thousand years longer than the principles that began western medicine. It can be argued that the current structure of western medicine is based on discoveries that date back only about one hundred years. I neither strive to argue against western medicine, nor contend we replace our system. Instead, I hope for more widespread realization that when western medicine no longer works, many reliable and helpful alternatives exist.

Consider what one exclusive physician shared. When cancer spread from one location, to another, my dad swallowed hard. His eyes glazed over with moisture. "I want to know how long," he bravely asserted.

"Do you want me to be honest," this very scientific, no-nonsense, renowned conventional oncologist asked.

"Of course," he replied, looking over at me as if wondering whether he should ask me to leave the room.

"I don't know," he answered. "This is not an attempt to frustrate you. If you want my scientific answer, it is 'I don't know.' The statistics I could offer you right now are based on data that is at least ten years old. Treatments have dramatically changed, but because of the research process, all I can offer is relatively ancient statistics."

My dad sat in silence. He had not asked for numbers any time before. He wanted an answer. Frustration filled the room.

"A more current estimate, based on world-wide data," the oncologist continued, seeking to appease my dad, who he could see wanted some indication, "indicates you have a fifty percent chance of living 6 months to 5 years. More specifically, about one in ten patients who come into my office with this diagnosis will be alive in 5 years. You could easily be the one. Every day you live beyond 5 years, your chances improve of us finding something that will work, of us finding a cure." Statistics are not accurately reflecting the fact that people given death sentences from doctors are living.

There is always hope. Check out Dr. Bernie Siegel's <u>Love, Medicine and Miracles</u>, Dr. Carl Simonton's <u>Getting Well Again</u>, Louise Hay's <u>You Can Heal Your</u>

Life, Michio Kushi's Macrobiotic Diet and The Cancer Prevention Diet, Dr. Ralph Moss' report on your type of cancer, Bridge of Hope by James Demers. Dr. Siegel has several books, meditation recordings in addition to his groups and conferences for exceptional cancer patients. Dr. Simonton holds conferences and retreats for patients throughout the world, with 30 years of groundbreaking work in the field of oncology. Psychologist Louise Hay suffered a death sentence alongside her ovarian cancer diagnosis, however cured herself and offers her method to the world with her best-selling books.

Michio Kushi his wife Aveline, world-renowned macrobiotic pioneers, founded the Kushi Institute, offering the macrobiotic way as a way of healing the body. In 2002, the Cancer Advisory Panel on Complimentary and Alternative Medicine (CAPCAM) studied six cases of cancer that the Kushi Institute presented to the National Cancer Institute (NCI). CAPCAM is comprised of both conventional and alternative professionals. Rigorous review examined medical records and macrobiotic evidence that the Kushi Institute provided, in hopes of determining if macrobiotics was the critical factor in the survival and recovery of these cancer patients. Six patients with initial diagnoses of stage IV metastatic cancer explained their case histories. Each patient fully recovered. Fifteen physicians and scientists called the evidence presented impressive and determined macrobiotics was worthy of further study, thus recommending the NCI fund a full clinical study on macrobiotics and cancer. While approving government funding for a clinical trial is wonderful news, consider the fact that this was the first unanimous agreement by the CAPCAM! James Demers book Bridge of Hope discusses the historical and treatment aspects of the herbal agent Essiac. These are only a few of the options available to you at any time on the cancer journey.

I remind myself daily of my dedication to endless hope by the prescription that remains taped to the side of my computer. A prescription slip from Dr. A, an endless giver of hope, who handed us the slip at the last appointment we ever had with him. This dedicated scientist looked sad, as he entered the room at 7pm to find my sister and I playing cards with my dad as we waited. He wrote the name of the drug down, as well as the company producing the drug, explaining, "If you can hold on until April 1st, we can start you on this promising drug." My dad held on until March 24th, ever hopeful. I continue to read up on the research being done in gastric cancer, and specifically the projects my dad's treatment team are involved in. Proton therapy has emerged, as well as the drug Dr. A wrote on that prescription slip. Hope is one thing cancer cannot take, it never dies.

Until the time comes inside where you feel a fight is no longer right and that the time for letting go has come, believe there are treatments, choices and hope. The only truly terminal part of cancer is hopelessness. As long as there is hope, there is life. I conclude by offering each person out there my heartfelt wishes for health, hope and, above all, adventure.

Chemo Bag

Chemotherapy and biological therapy administration for my dad consisted of at least 6-hour days to as many as 168 hour stays. It was a long, drawn out, tedious process. To ameliorate the process, I created a chemo bag. Using a canvas bag, I tossed in a variety of ingredients mentioned within the chapters of this book to make the day as pleasant as possible.

Create a Chemo Bag Containing:
1. Mints/Gum
2. Lotion (the dry hospital environment dries the skin)
3. Antibacterial hand rub
4. Acupressure wrist bands
5. A hand held massager
6. DVD's and/or videos
7. A DVD/video player, laptop or portable DVD player
8. A microwave bean pack
9. A mini pill box with a couple pain pills
10. Bags incase of vomiting
11. Latex or woven gloves
12. A surgical face mask
13. A notebook and a pen
14. Possibly the personal question and answer diaries I recommended a patient filling in (if the patient feels well enough to write during chemo).
15. An iPod
16. A 3x5 card with all drugs, vitamins, supplements, herbs and over-the-counter medications listed.
17. Antibacterial mouth wash
18. Bottled Water
19. Ear Plugs

20. List of all the doctors' phone numbers (if they're not all programmed in your phone)

Some other ideas incase you have room....
- Tea bags
- List of 5 closest pharmacy's phone numbers (if they're not all programmed in your phone)
- Books (Lance Armstrong provides a particularly good read in that environment!)
- Small soft blanket
- Soft socks

Cancer First Aid Kit

A cancer first aid kit is necessary to increase a feeling of ease at home. Have the items most likely to be needed on hand in case they become necessary. Find a basket, plastic box or container, designate a drawer or shelf and prepare your cancer first aid kit before it becomes necessary. Include:

1. Bandages – a variety pack with small to large sizes
2. Betadine Solution
3. Rubbing Alcohol
4. Hydrogen Peroxide
5. Antibacterial topical ointment
6. A reliable thermometer
7. Back-up supply of disposable thermometers
8. Cotton Balls
9. Cotton Swabs
10. Latex Gloves
11. Blood pressure monitor

Cancer Materials and Gifts

Cancer storms into life, often turning up everything in its path, creating a treacherous, unexplored path for families. One day I was picking out nice shirts and ties for father's day; then by the time my dad's birthday arrived, I was searching for useful gifts in the face of cancer. Here are a plethora of gift ideas for any cancer patient in your life.

1. Journals or spiral notebooks with lined paper.
2. Large, 2-3 inch, 3-ring notebook.
3. Business card pages, usually made of poly material that can go in the binder. Mine hold up to 20 cards a page.
4. Scrap booking materials. Visit the nearest craft store or scrapbook specialty store.
5. Natural and researched multivitamins.
6. Plastic container/bowl/trash can to act as a vomit receptacle (consider buying several based on your individual needs).
7. Camera
8. Video camera
9. Store of extra toothbrushes
10. Pill Boxes
11. Anti-nausea acupressure wrist bands
12. Bead packs (for all parts of the body)
13. Egg crates
14. Shower Chair
15. DVD's and Videos (comedies in particular)
16. Bags to put in the car (incase of nausea)
17. Vibrating chair cover
18. Soft Blankets
19. Soft Socks

20. Soft Slippers
21. Mint or lavender candles
22. Natural and gentle bath products like shower gel and bubble bath
23. Natural and gentle lotions – especially those with mint, spearmint, peppermint, lavender or chamomile.
24. Books like those from Lance Armstrong and Dr. Bernie Siegel.
25. A DVD and Video combo player to take to the hospital, or a portable DVD player.

References

Balch, P.A. (2006). Prescription for Nutritional Healing: A Practical A-to-Z Reference to
    Drug-Free Remedies Using Vitamins, Minerals, Herbs and Food Supplements (4th
    ed.). New York, NY: Penguin Group.

Brooks, M. (Director). (1974). Blazing Saddles [Film]. Burbank, CA: Warner Brothers.

Countryman, J. (1996). A Father's Legacy. Nashville, TN: Thomas Nelson.

Countryman, J. (2007). A Grandparent's Legacy. Nashville, TN: Thomas Nelson.

Countryman, J. (2007). A Mother's Legacy. Nashville, TN: Thomas Nelson.

Cousins, N. (2005). Anatomy of an Illness as Perceived by the Patient. New York, NY:
    Norton, W.W. & Company, Inc.

Cromie, W.J. (2002). Meditation changes temperatures: Mind controls body in extreme experiments. *Harvard University Gazette*. Retrieved April 30, 2002, http://www.hno.harvard.edu/gazette/2002/04.18/09-tummo.html.

Demers, J. (2003). Bridge of Hope. Ontario: Bracebridge Publishing.

Hay, L. (1984). You Can Heal Your Life. Carlsbad, CA: Hay House.

Tremaine, J. (Director). (2002). <u>Jackass: The Movie</u> [Film]. Hollywood, CA: Paramount
      Pictures.

Kessler, D. (2000). <u>The Needs of the Dying.</u> New York, NY: Harper Collins Publishers.

Kübler-Ross, E. (1997). <u>On Death and Dying.</u> New York, NY: Simon and Schuster Publishers.

Kübler-Ross, E., & Kessler, D. (2001). <u>Life Lessons: Two Experts on Death and Dying</u>
      <u>Teach us About the Mysteries of Life and Living</u>. New York, NY: Simon and Schuster Publishers.

Kübler-Ross, E., & Kessler, D. (2005). <u>On Grief and Grieving: Finding the Meaning of</u>
      <u>Grief Through the Five Stages of Loss.</u> New York, NY: Scribner Publishers.

Kushi, M., & Kushi, A. (1993). <u>Macrobiotic Diet.</u> Tokyo: Japan Publications.

Kushi, M., & Jack, A. (1993). <u>The Cancer Prevention Diet.</u> England: St. Martin's Press.

Siegel, B. <u>Love, Medicine and Miracles.</u> Minneapolis, MN: Quill House Publishers,
      1986.

Siegel, B. <u>Peace, Love and Healing.</u> Minneapolis, MN: Quill House Publishers, 1998.

Siegel, B. (Speaker). (2004). <u>Getting Ready</u> [Audiocassette]. Carlsbad, CA: Hay House.

Siegel, B. (Speaker). (2003). Healing Meditations
[Audiocassette]. Carlsbad, CA: Hay
House.

Siegel, B. (Speaker). (2004). Meditations for Difficult
Times [Audiocassette]. Carlsbad,
CA: Hay House.

Siegel, B. (Speaker). (1998). Meditations for Enhancing
Your Immune System:
Strengthen Your Body's Ability to Heal
[Audiocassette]. Carlsbad, CA: Hay
House.

Siegel, B. (Speaker). (2006). Meditations for Finding the
Key to Good Health
[Audiocassette]. Carlsbad, CA: Hay House.

Siegel, B. (Speaker). (2004). Meditations for Morning and
Evening [Audiocassette].
Carlsbad, CA: Hay House.

Siegel, B. (Speaker). (2004). Medications for Overcoming
Life's Stresses and Strains
[Audiocassette]. Carlsbad, CA: Hay House.

Siegel, B. (Speaker). (2004). Medications for Peace of
Mind [Audiocassette]. Carlsbad,
CA: Hay House.

Simonton, C.O., Matthews-Simonton, Stephanie &
Creighton, James. (1992). Getting
Well Again. New York: Bantam Books.

www.ingramcontent.com/pod-product-compliance
Lightning Source LLC
Chambersburg PA
CBHW030019290326
41934CB00005B/405